REPRODUCTIVE
ENDOCRINOLOGY
AND
INFERTILITY

REPRODUCTIVE ENDOCRINOLOGY AND INFERTILITY

CURRENT TRENDS AND DEVELOPMENTS

edited by

Seang Lin Tan
McGill University and McGill University Health Centre
Montreal, Quebec, Canada

Togas Tulandi
McGill University
Montreal, Quebec, Canada

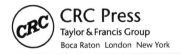

CRC Press
Taylor & Francis Group
Boca Raton London New York

CRC Press is an imprint of the
Taylor & Francis Group, an **informa** business

CRC Press
Taylor & Francis Group
6000 Broken Sound Parkway NW, Suite 300
Boca Raton, FL 33487-2742

First issued in paperback 2019

© 2003 by Taylor & Francis Group, LLC
CRC Press is an imprint of Taylor & Francis Group, an Informa business

No claim to original U.S. Government works

ISBN-13: 978-0-8247-0844-3 (hbk)
ISBN-13: 978-0-367-39571-1 (pbk)

**Visit the Taylor & Francis Web site at
http://www.taylorandfrancis.com**

**and the CRC Press Web site at
http://www.crcpress.com**

Preface

Because reproductive medicine is a rapidly evolving science, dogma that is widely accepted one year might not be applicable the next. Since 1996, the Department of Obstetrics and Gynecology at McGill University has organized an annual international symposium on reproductive endocrinology and infertility with a stellar cast of world-renowned speakers who have addressed many of the latest advances in the field. This book is a compilation of key topics that have been covered at the annual meetings and reflects the latest thinking in contraception, hormone replacement therapy, assisted reproductive technologies, and reproductive surgery.

The contributors are physicians and scientists who are leaders in the field. Michael Cho, Judi Marraccini, and Brian Little review a topic of great importance to women as they approach the menopausal transition, namely, the choice and risks associated with various forms of contraception. In the past few years, a number of oral contraceptive formulations have been introduced that contain markedly lower hormonal doses. Sally Perlman and Joseph Sanfilippo discuss the indications for use of these ultralow-dose oral contraceptive preparations in comparison with conventional oral contraceptives. Although androgen therapy for menopausal women has been used for many years, it remains an area of considerable debate and there is no consensus regarding its use. Camille Sylvestre and Morrie Gelfand, who have long championed the use of androgen treatment for menopausal women, discuss this controversial topic. Although the benefits of short-term hormone replacement therapy in symptomatic women are well recognized, the use of long-term hormone replacement therapy to prevent osteoporosis and cardiovascular disease has been increasingly challenged over the past 2 years. In part, this is due to the underlying concern about any association between hormone replacement therapy and cancer. Elene Strates and Charles Coddington elegantly review this topical subject. Richard Kremer and David Goltzman discuss the plethora of alternative therapies for the prevention of osteoporosis that have recently become available.

Chapters 6, 7, and 8 focus on recent advances in assisted reproductive technologies. Although in vitro fertilization is a very successful treatment, its use is associated with a risk of ovarian hyperstimulation syndrome, and the only reliable way to prevent this complication is to avoid use of this treatment. In the past few years, a number of studies have indicated that in vitro maturation of oocytes may be an appropriate alternative treatment for selected patients. Timothy Child and Seang Lin Tan discuss how this technology can be optimally used for infertility treatment today. In the past decade, a few hundred babies have been born after preimplantation genetic diagnosis. Asangla Ao discusses recent advances in this fascinating area. Hang Yin, Roger Gosden, and Ahmad Kamal Abdul-Jalil review the state of the art in human oocyte cryopreservation.

The last three chapters deal with surgical aspects of reproductive medicine. Carla Roberts and John Rock review the treatment of uterine anomalies, and Mazen Bisharah and Togas Tulandi lucidly delineate the principles of practical management of ectopic pregnancy. Pelvic pain afflicts a large number of women and in the last chapter Christopher Sutton discusses the use of laparoscopic surgery for the management of this dehabilitating condition.

In the past decade, there has been an explosion of advances in the field of clinical reproductive medicine. This book focuses on many aspects of treatment and care in which these advances have touched the lives of many women seeking help from their physicians. This book is valuable for both physicians in training and practicing obstetricians and gynecologists. We are grateful to our contributors for their comprehensive and authoritative reviews, which we hope you will find both stimulating and beneficial to your clinical practice.

Seang Lin Tan
Togas Tulandi

Contents

Preface   *iii*

Contributors   *ix*

1. Contraception for Women Over Age 40 Years   1
   Michael M. Cho, Judi Marraccini, and A. Brian Little

2. Ultralow-Dose Oral Contraception   23
   Sally E. Perlman and Joseph S. Sanfilippo

3. Hormone Replacement Therapy and the Role of
   Androgens   39
   Camille Sylvestre and Morrie M. Gelfand

4. Hormone Replacement Therapy and Cancer   57
   Elene Strates and Charles C. Coddington

5. Alternatives to Hormonal Replacement Therapy for
   Prevention of Osteoporosis   81
   Richard Kremer and David Goltzman

6. In Vitro Maturation of Oocytes for Infertility
Treatment   109
Timothy J. Child and Seang Lin Tan

7. Preimplantation Genetic Diagnosis   133
Asangla Ao

8. Human Oocyte Cryopreservation   165
*Hang Yin, Roger G. Gosden, and Ahmad Kamal
Abdul-Jalil*

9. Treatment of Uterine Anomalies   195
Carla P. Roberts and John A. Rock

10. Practical Management of Ectopic Pregnancy   225
Mazen Bisharah and Togas Tulandi

11. Laparoscopic Surgery for Pelvic Pain   245
Christopher Sutton

Index   *285*

Contributors

Ahmad Kamal Abdul-Jalil, M.Sc. Department of Obstetrics and Gynecology, McGill University and McGill University Health Centre, Montreal, Quebec, Canada

Asangla Ao, Ph.D. Department of Obstetrics and Gynecology, McGill University and McGill University Health Centre, Montreal, Quebec, Canada

Mazen Bisharah, M.D., F.R.C.S.C. Department of Obstetrics and Gynecology, McGill University and McGill University Health Centre, Montreal, Quebec, Canada

Timothy J. Child, M.A., M.B.B.S., M.R.C.O.G. Department of Obstetrics and Gynecology, John Radcliffe Hospital, Oxford, England

Michael M. Cho, M.D. Department of Obstetrics, Gynecology, and Women's Health, University of Medicine and Dentistry of New Jersey and New Jersey Medical School, Newark, New Jersey, U.S.A.

Charles C. Coddington, M.D. Department of Obstetrics and Gynecology, Denver Health Medical Center and University of Colorado, Denver, Colorado, U.S.A.

Morrie M. Gelfand, M.D., F.R.C.S.(C), F.A.C.S., F.A.C.O.G.   Department of Obstetrics and Gynecology, Sir Mortimer B. Davis Jewish General Hospital and McGill University, Montreal, Quebec, Canada

David Goltzman, M.D.   Department of Obstetrics and Gynecology, McGill University and McGill University Health Centre, Montreal, Quebec, Canada

Roger G. Gosden, Ph.D., D.Sc.   Department of Obstetrics and Gynecology, The Jones Institute for Reproductive Medicine, Norfolk, Virginia, U.S.A.

Richard Kremer, M.D., Ph.D., F.R.C.P.(C)   Department of Obstetrics and Gynecology, McGill University and McGill University Health Centre, Montreal, Quebec, Canada

A. Brian Little, M.D., F.R.C.S.(C)   Department of Obstetrics, Gynecology, and Women's Health, University of Medicine and Dentistry of New Jersey and New Jersey Medical School, Newark, New Jersey, U.S.A.

Judi Marraccini, B.A.   Department of Obstetrics, Gynecology, and Women's Health, University of Medicine and Dentistry of New Jersey and New Jersey Medical School, Newark, New Jersey, U.S.A.

Sally E. Perlman, M.D.   Department of Obstetrics, The University of Louisville School of Medicine, Louisville, Kentucky, U.S.A.

Carla P. Roberts, M.D., Ph.D.   Department of Obstetrics and Gynecology, Emory University School of Medicine, Atlanta, Georgia, U.S.A.

John A. Rock, M.D.   Department of Obstetrics and Gynecology, Emory University School of Medicine, Atlanta, Georgia, U.S.A.

Joseph S. Sanfilippo, M.D., M.B.A. Department of Obstetrics, Gynecology, and Reproductive Sciences, The University of Pittsburgh School of Medicine, and Vice Chairman, Reproductive Sciences, Magee-Women's Hospital, Pittsburgh, Pennsylvania, U.S.A.

Elene Strates, M.D. Department of Obstetrics and Gynecology, Denver Health Medical Center and University of Colorado, Denver, Colorado, U.S.A.

Christopher Sutton, M.A., M.B.B.,Ch(Cantab), F.R.C.O.G. Department of Obstetrics and Gynecology, Royal Surrey County Hospital and University of Surrey, Guilford, Surrey, England

Camille Sylvestre, M.D., F.R.C.S.(C) Department of Obstetrics and Gynecology, McGill University and McGill University Health Centre, Montreal, Quebec, Canada

Seang Lin Tan, M.B.B.S., F.R.C.O.G., F.R.C.S.(C) Department of Obstetrics and Gynecology, McGill University and McGill University Health Centre, Montreal, Quebec, Canada

Togas Tulandi, M.D., F.R.C.S.C. Department of Obstetrics and Gynecology, McGill University, Montreal, Quebec, Canada

Hang Yin, Ph.D. Department of Obstetrics and Gynecology, The Jones Institute for Reproductive Medicine, Norfolk, Virginia, U.S.A.

REPRODUCTIVE
ENDOCRINOLOGY
AND
INFERTILITY

1

Contraception for Women Over Age 40 Years

Michael M. Cho, Judi Marraccini, and A. Brian Little
University of Medicine and Dentistry of New Jersey and New Jersey Medical School, Newark, New Jersey, U.S.A.

Am I still likely to get pregnant? Is the menopause at 40? How can I tell when it comes?

What about infections? I don't and surely my husband doesn't, but he might? And I could . . .

What about the birth control pills and heart disease, or hypertension? I have diabetes.

Should I still have intercourse at my age?

What about shots? Skin patches? What's Norplant?

What do my hot flashes mean? Can I no longer get pregnant?

I had a breast removed because of cancer and I still have periods. Can I get pregnant? Will my cancer get worse if I take oral contraceptives?

I had chemotherapy for lymphoma. Should I use contraception?

Women are said to live longer, be healthier, and continue to have sex later in life than in previous times. The classical view of "Dad and mom surely don't have sex any longer," has been replaced somewhat by the view that most people as they grow older are still doing all those things we used to believe were restricted to our younger years, and we can still do so; and we now say, "Perhaps even mother does . . ." and so now we can . . .

With the aging of the population, more attention is paid to advancing years; as we become a nation of advertisements and publicists, the activities of the older elements of the population become the focus of study for marketing purposes. However, in many physicians' offices, the usual authoritative figure has been slow to be replaced, and the subject of sex and contraception is not usually broached spontaneously. When it is, all the details of sexuality are not always exchanged as simply as symptoms of heart disease, for example. However, if the physician begins with a knowledge that sexuality is an integral part of women's lives after the age of 40 years, and that even those women whose husbands may not be active or satisfying will often seek their own emotional release with someone else, the physician can advise more realistically, even in the face of the frequent comment, "I don't need that advice!"

I. FERTILITY AND FECUNDITY IN WOMEN OVER THE AGE OF 40 YEARS

Some women still believe that their ability to conceive vanishes at the age of 40 years, although this is not true (Table 1 [1,2]). The births by older women in the United States consistently decrease after the age of 35 years, so that the birth rate at 35–39 years is 36.0 births per 1000 women and 0.3 births per 1000 women between the ages of 45 and 49 years. This represents approximately 408,000 births at the earlier age and 78,000 births after age 40 years [3]. These rates continue to decrease in the recent health statistics. It also is little appreciated that having a baby as late as the end of the fourth decade of life is associated with a number of costs and risks (including malformation). The incidences of disease, particularly chronic diseases, increase and conse-

Table 1 Projected Fertility Rates by Race, 1998–2010 (Live Births per 1000 Women)

Age (years)	All races	White	Black	American Indian	Asian/ Pacific	Islander Hispanic
40–44	5.7–5.9	5.4–5.6	5.4–5.3	6.0–6.0	10.3–10.3	10.8–10.8
45–49	0.3–0.3	0.2–0.2	0.3–0.2	0.3–0.3	1.0–1.0	0.6–0.6

"Demographic statistics of fertility rates do not necessarily reflect natural fertility, but depend on social trends in child bearing and contraceptive use." (*Source*: Ref 1.) Those who do not use contraceptives are reported to have an average age of 40.9 years at their last delivery.
Source: Ref. 5.

quently, maternal mortality rises from less than 19.6 per 100,000 live births (age 35–39 years) to 258 per 100,000 at the older ages (45+ years) [4]. This rate is almost 0.3 per 100 live births, which is a sizeable and threatening statistic.

It has been said that abortion should be the backup for failed contraception. It appears that this might even be more applicable for women who are older than 40 years. Although the number of abortions (number of abortions per 1000 total abortions *and* live births) increases from 216 at 35–39 years of age to almost 301 for women over the age of 40 years, [5] the number of live births is much less, and thus abortions are not so prevalent at these later years as the figures might appear to indicate at first glance. Of these pregnancies after age 40 years, abortions accounted for some of those resulting from failed contraception, which range between 0 for sterilization (female) and 2.9 for condom per 1000 women-years [2]. However, at older ages, the failed method range is wide and provocative when related to each other and more so when compared to values of younger women. Abortion is not the method of choice for contraception at any age, and even less so after age 40 years.

The apparent natural decline in fertility (Table 1) and fecundity (the average monthly probability of conception) has often been noted. Toward the end of the 1960s, when the "baby boomers" came of age and women began to be more recognized in the professions and in the workplace, there appeared a fear that women who put off developing their family might not be able to have as many babies as they would like after the age of 30 years. A classic review of that time concluded that although ". . . infecundity is a problem . . . attention should be directed toward disease and not distorted by an exaggerated impression of the normal biological effects of aging. The risk of being unable to bear a child . . . increases with age from about 5–6% at 20–24 to at most 16% when she is 30–35." These conclusions were based on the review of data from disparate places and eras from Switzerland, England, Germany, and Quebec, through the years 1600, 1800, and 1950, where the studies have been of normal married populations [6].

II. CLASSICAL CONTRACEPTIVE REQUIREMENTS

Ideal contraceptives have always been measured on the classical elements of efficacy, safety, tolerability, reversibility, coital independence, and protection from sexually transmitted disease. Any of the classical considerations may outweigh other considerations and make it possible and advisable to prescribe a method which does not necessarily meet all the criteria expressed. For example, among all methods (Table 2 [7]), one of the best and most used forms of contraception after the age of 40 years, is sterilization. This obviously does not fulfill the criteria of reversibility. There is a belief in the community that "tubes may be untied," which is regrettable. Although this misconception derived from original "tying" of the fallopian tubes with suture, sterilization should always be undertaken as permanent and irreversible. Otherwise, there are too many caveats for patients to cling to, and results of tubal reanastomosis (which even in the best of situations is a far from perfect procedure) deteriorate, depending on how much of the fallopian tubes were left, and in what state they were, left (e.g., postcauterization).

III. PERMANENT METHODS (STERILIZATION)

Among women over the age of 40 years desiring contraception, more than half rely on tubal sterilization. The overall cumulative failure rate is 1.3 %. Failure rates vary by method (Table 3) [4]: with age over 40

Table 2 Contraceptive Status of Women (%)[a]

	All	25–34 (years)	35–44 (years)
Surgically sterile	24.8	22.4	46.8
Pregnant or postpartum	4.6	6.9	1.3
Seeking pregnancy	4.0	6.2	3.5
Among nonusers, no inter- course last months	6.2	5.3	6.5
Pill	17.3	23.7	6.3
IUD	0.5	0.6	0.8
Diaphragm	1.2	1.2	2.0
Condom	13.1	15.0	10.7
Periodic abstinence (natural family planning)	1.7	2.1	2.2
Withdrawal	2.0	2.3	1.9
Other (Depo—implants, etc.)	3.9	4.2	2.1

[a] Other omitted categories bring the total to 100%.

Table 3 Failure Rates After 2 Years per 100 Women-Years

	Age (years)	
	(25–34)	(>35)
Oral contraceptives	0.38	0.23
Progestin	2.50	0.50
Intrauterine copper devices	3.10	0.60
Diaphragm	5.50	2.80
Condom	6.00	2.90
Sterilization (M)	0.08	0.00
Sterilization (F)	0.45	0.08

Motivation determines ideal versus typical failure rate; thus, actual rates may be optimal for older, more motivated women.
Source: Ref. 4.

years, the failure rate is lower. In addition, a noncontraceptive benefit of tubal sterilization includes a lower risk of ovarian cancer [8].

Among married perimenopausal women, partner vasectomy is the second most common contraceptive method. Vasectomy carries a relatively modest surgical risk for men, and no significant physical side effects have been documented. Reanastomosis is difficult (60% success), and spermiogenesis is reduced with significant delay. There is no significant increased risk of prostate cancer, myocardial infarction, angina pectoris, coronary vascular diseases, or stroke [8].

IV. SYSTEMIC HORMONAL CONTRACEPTIVES

A. Oral Contraceptives

There is no increased incidence of myocardial infarction or stroke among healthy, older (>40 years) nonsmokers taking oral contraceptives (OCs) containing less than 50 μg estrogen [9]. Oral contraceptives may be the contraceptive of choice for women over 40 years old because of resulting regular menses, the positive effect on bone mineral density, the reduction of vasomotor symptoms, and the reduced risk of endometrial and ovarian cancer, without increased risk of breast cancer [10,11].

The mortality of nonsmokers using OCs is lower than for barrier method users because of the higher mortality associated with pregnancies either terminated or going to term in association with barrier failures.

Oral contraceptives with and estrogen dose of 50 μg or less are not associated with an increase in cardiovascular mortality after the age of 35 years. The known increased risk is associated with smokers or those with cardiac risk factors [12].

Stroke is rare in women of childbearing age. Excluding hypertension, the odds ratio for ischemic or hemorrhagic stroke with current oral contraceptive use were not substantially higher for older women than for younger women [12]. The adjusted odds ratio for all types of stroke among current OC users was 1.16 (95% confidence interval [95% CI], 0.72–1.88). In the same study, 96% of current users used less than 50 µg of estrogen [13] A Danish study [14] confirmed that the relative risk of ischemic stroke among users of low-estrogen OCs compared to non-users is not more than 2.5.

There is no increase in breast cancer and an actual decrease of 4–50% in risk of endometrial and ovarian cancer in former users [11]. A slight increased risk of thromboembolic disease is present regardless of smoking status. New progestational agents (so-called "third-generation OCs"), by eliminating lipid, carbohydrate, and other metabolic changes associated with currently used progestins, show a small reduction in the already low overall risks of the nonsmoking older women [15,16].

V. LONG-TERM SYSTEMIC HORMONAL CONTRACEPTIVES

A. Implants

Long-term methods such as the levonorgestrel implant system, depot medroxyprogesterone acetate (DMPA), the levonorgestrel-releasing intrauterine device (IUD), and the copper-T 380A IUD all provide reversible contraception with protection that is essentially equal to that provided by permanent methods.

Norplant and the two-rod levonorgestrel implant system are highly efficacious, and have failure rates of <1% [17]. The major disadvantage of using implants for a woman who is approaching menopause is the abnormalities observed in menstrual bleeding. The pattern of bleeding may make it difficult to distinguish physiological changes expected at menopause from pathological changes which cause similar genital tract bleeding. By far the most common side effect for women of any age using contraceptive implants is the affected change in menstrual pattern. This tends to occur frequently during the first 6–9 months of use, but usually stabilizes by the end of the first year. A positive aspect of the progestin is the beneficial effect on the endometrium, counteracting the effects of unopposed estrogen on the uterus in this age group. Side effects include headache, vaginal discharge, weight gain, acne, pelvic pain, and mood alterations.

B. Contraceptive Patch

A sustained-release device, the contraceptive patch provides daily steroid doses and maximum concentration determined by the size of the patch [18]. Evra® (a contraceptive patch) is equivalent to the lowest-dose oral contraceptives (150 μg of 17-deacetyl-norgestimate and 20 μg of ethinyl estradiol). Worn 3 out of 4 weeks (21 days out of 28), the patch has the advantage of being self-administered once a week [19]. The side effects and limitations are similar to those of low-dose oral contraceptives.

C. Injectable

Monthly combined hormonal injectable contraceptive (Lunelle®, containing 5 mg estradiol cypionate and 25 mg medroxyprogesterone acetate) has the same advantage and limitation profile as those of combined oral contraceptives. It is highly effective (failure rates of only 2 per 100 women-years) [20,21]. The return to fertility is rapid after discontinuation of treatment [22], however, menorrhagia and dysmenorrhea limit its use [23].

A major disadvantage of using Depo-Provera (DMPA) is the prolonged delay of return of regular menses and fertility (up to 20 months [24]). This makes DMPA a poor choice for older women, who might be attracted to this method for pregnancy spacing or other reasons.

VI. LONG-TERM NONSYSTEMIC CONTRACEPTIVES

A. Intrauterine Devices

Both intrauterine copper and progestin-releasing intrauterine devices are appropriate for perimenopausal women. Abnormal bleeding is common among some women who experience ovarian dysfunction perimenopause. The nature of those changes may affect IUD selection. Copper IUDs will tend to increase bleeding, particularly during the first few cycles, whereas progestin-releasing devices decrease total menstrual blood loss but may prolong the menstrual period of light bleeding. Perimenopausal women who are experiencing menorrhagia that is not attributable to any obvious pathological causes may benefit from a progesterone-releasing IUD [25].

A copper IUD is appropriate for use in women with the following medical conditions: cardiovascular diseases, including hypertension with vascular and renal complications, and dyslipidemia; hematologic disorders such as thromboembolism; liver disease; diabetes mellitus (with vascular disease); neurologic conditions; and psychiatric disorders.

The only medical conditions in which IUDs are contraindicated are those that make women more susceptible to infection (leukemia, intravenous drug abuse, acquired immunodeficiency syndrome [AIDS]); and diseases (e.g., hematological) or medications that lead to profuse uterine bleeding; conditions that distort the uterine cavity; and Wilson's disease. In the latter, specifically the copper IUD is contraindicated.

VII. BARRIER CONTRACEPTIVES

The male condom is the most popular barrier contraceptive among women (30–40% incidence) of the 40–45-year-old age group. The main advantages in this age group are the absence of pharmacological metabolic risk, low cost, sexually transmitted disease (STD) protection, and availability without prescription. The increased compliance and lower fecundity of mature women partially offset the higher failure rate generally quoted for condoms. However, condom use may influence male impotence and lead to ejaculatory difficulty. The protection obtained by use of the condom against STDs cannot be overemphasized.

The diaphragm is used by 9–13% of women ages 40–44 years. However, the effectiveness of this method may be reduced by uterine descensus and vaginal relaxation. The cervical cap avoids the problem of proper vaginal placement, but few women, primary care physicians, or specialty physicians have been trained to fit caps properly.

VIII. CONTRACEPTIVE CHOICES IN WOMEN WITH MEDICAL AND GYNECOLOGICAL PROBLEMS

A. Diabetes

Combined Hormonal Contraceptives

As women get older, many gain weight and may develop diabetes. Non-insulin-dependent diabetes mellitus (type II) becomes manifest particularly among patients over the age of 40 years. The choice of contraception must reflect due consideration of the risk of the OC on the disease; and against it, the risk of becoming pregnant with diabetes. Women with diabetes have a higher complication rate during pregnancy, a higher rate of miscarriage, and an increased risk for fetal congenital malformation.

There is no present evidence that the use of combined hormonal contraception adversely affects the development or progression of diabetes. There is no increased risk of diabetes among the current users of contraceptive pills (risk ratio [RR] 0.8, 95% CI, 0.49–1.32), even among those who had used the pill for a long time. Similarly, there is no association between diabetes and former users of the pill (RR 0.82, 95% CI, 0.59–1.13) [26]. The use of combination oral contraceptives among young women with insulin-dependent diabetes mellitus does not pose an additional risk for the development of early diabetic retinopathy and/or nephropathy [27]. Neither the current nor past use, nor number of years of use of oral contraceptives, is associated with the severity of retinopathy, hypertension, or an increased level of glycosylated hemoglobin in women with type I diabetes [28].

Progestin-Only Contraceptives

Subdermal implant of levonorgestrel (Norplant) appears to alter carbohydrate metabolism. Although such alterations are not clinically significant in normal women, its use in diabetic women warrants close medical follow-up [29].

Among women susceptible to developing diabetes, the use of a progestin-only contraceptive appears to affect them adversely. Although progestin-only oral contraceptives are associated with an increased risk of diabetes in breast-feeding young Latinas with recent gestational diabetes mellitus (GDM), no increased risk of type II diabetes was observed among those who had a GDM history while taking low-dose combination oral contraceptive as compared to controls [30].

Nonhormonal Contraception

A copper-containing intrauterine device appears to be a good choice for diabetic women. The continuation rate and the events leading to termination of use of the IUDs were comparable in the diabetic (type I, insulin-dependent diabetes mellitus (IDDM]) to nondiabetic groups during the first 3 years of use [31]. There were no increased incidences of pregnancy or pelvic infection among diabetic women as compared to nondiabetic women [32].

B.   Cardiovascular Disease/Hypertensive Disorder

Lipid Disorders

Perhaps there are still those members of the general public that do not know about cholesterol and heart disease, and there may still be a few that do not realize that the estrogen in the pill is the same generic substance as that in the estrogen replacement taken postmenopause. However, there is considerable confusion as to when the menopause occurs, when one should start estrogen replacement (if at all), and whether estrogen of the contraceptive pill is of any benefit in the years after age 40, before estrogen replacement is usually prescribed. Finally, estrogen's effects on lipids and heart disease in women is uncertain. Simply stated, dyslipidemia is the excessive entry into the blood stream of lipoproteins, a reduced removal of them, or a combination of both caused by altered metabolism or genetic factors. Most of the problems seen are those of the altered metabolism as a result of the dietary habits of those susceptible to such alterations. Most practitioners are familiar with the obese, hypertensive patient with a family history of diabetes who after the age of 40 years develops hypercholesterolemia and elevated low-density lipoprotein (LDL), who is not inclined to take OCs, or for some economic reason cannot afford them. The easiest course is to prescribe a barrier contraceptive and treat the excess cholesterol independently. However, OCs may be beneficial for this group, because estrogen will lower LDL and increase circulating high-density lipoprotein (HDL) (which is beneficial to the risk for heart disease) and reduce cholesterol. The moderate increase of triglyceride associated with OCs does not appear to affect the risk for cardiovascular disease [33]. In all cases, healthy diet and lifestyle will prevent coronary heart disease and reduce abnormal lipidemia, and should be reinforced [34]. The incidence of myocardial infarction is not increased among healthy, non-smoking, older women (>40 years) taking OCs [9].

Hypertension

Hypertension is commonly encountered among patients who request OCs after the age of 40 years. Such women should be taking medication to maintain the blood pressure at reasonably normal levels. Oral contraceptives are safe to prescribe to such patients, providing they have no vascular and/or renal complications of hypertension, and if their diastolic blood pressure while taking medication is maintained below 100 mm Hg. Oral contraceptives per se do increase blood pressure, but only a small amount, and mortality is not materially increased [35]. Blood pressure should be checked 6 weeks after the patients taking OCs.

C. Osteoporosis

Of the 35–50 % cortical and trabecular bone mass measured as bone mineral density (BMD) lost over a woman's lifetime, about 10% may be lost in the perimenopause (5 years premenopause). This can be compared to the postmenopause loss of 1.5–3.0% per year (mostly trabecular).

Continuing use of OCs has been shown to result in an optimal increase in total body BMD measured premenopause in the lumbar forearm and total body. Others have shown no relationship between OCs and BMD (ages 45–49 years). Perimenopausal women can be expected to exhibit a decreased BMD with a history of more than 10 years of taking OCs [36].

Bone-sparing effects of estrogen may not be met at the OC content of 20 µg/day, because there is actually a net loss at 15 µg/day and net gain at 25 µg/day. Progestational agents, particularly norethindrone, may exert positive effects on BMD [36]. Therefore, OCs with norethindrone seem to be indicated, and OCs with 25–35 µg of estrogen plus norethindrone may be best.

D. Hematological Diseases

Sickle Cell

Patients with homozygous sickle cell disease (SS) apparently have an inhibition of in vivo sickling during DMPA treatment. Painful crises are less frequent during DMPA treatment, accompanied by rising fetal hemoglobin (Hb F), total hemoglobin, and red cell mass, count, and survival rate. The improvement may not be entirely the result of DMPA; another study suggested that reduced pain is not associated with improved hemoglobin parameters [37]. In fact, good medical treatment of control subjects in such studies may have resulted in an almost equivalent reduction in pain [38].

E. Cancers

Breast Cancer

Frequently, treatment for breast cancer will induce menopause. However it has been recently shown that estrogen replacement has no adverse impact on recurrence and mortality. Taking into consideration the presence of normal menstrual bleeding, the hormone dependence of the tumor and stage of its spread there may be an indication for the cautious administration of OCs or estrogen replacement which may be important for such women over the age of 40 years [39].

F. Neurological Disorders

Migraine Headaches

The exact cause of headaches is difficult for most physicians to diagnose and headaches are frequent complaints of women over the age of 40 years. Most are tension headaches [40]. The symptoms of some women with migraine get better, while others get worse. Most migraines in women taking OCs occur in the last week of pills (28-day packs) containing no hormone. The women with classic migraine with aura is associated with a four-fold increase in ischemic stroke, whereas those without aura have been shown to have a three-fold increase that was not significant [41]. Although those with a history of stroke were shown to have an increased risk of six times compared to those not using OCs (without a history of stroke), this result was not significant. Among those women who smoked and had a history of migraine, there was a 34-fold increased risk of stroke. Therefore, for women with migraine, who smoke or not, it is safer to prescribe progestin-only pills, IUD, or barrier contraceptives. Careful follow-up should be maintained in those women prescribed OCs if they have auras, history of stroke, neurological signs, or are smokers, when it is impossible to find an alternative.

Seizure Disorders

Depot medroxyprogesterone acetate should be considered in women with history of seizure disorder because DMPA may contribute to a reduced seizure rate [42]. There is no evidence that epileptic seizures are exacerbated by oral contraceptives [43]. However, some antiepileptic drugs (Table 4 [44]) can decrease the efficacy of low-dose combined oral contraceptives.

Table 4 Antiepileptic Medications that Can Affect OC Effectiveness

Anticonvulsants	
Do not reduce steroid level	Do reduce steroid levels
Valporic acid	Barbiturates
Gabapentin	Phenytoin
Lamotrigine	Carbamazepine
Tiagabine	Felbamate
	Vigabatrin

Source: Ref. 44.

Alzheimer's Disease

Whether estrogen has beneficial effects on cognition is controversial, and it has been debated for almost 50 years. Although results suggest the improvement of verbal memory and attention, the effects on cognition postmenopause are conflicting [45]. Selective estrogen receptor modulators (SERMS) have yet to be shown to have such an effect [46]. Unsettled is also the question whether OCs continued after age 40 years through the perimenopause contribute to any protective effect.

G. Mentally III and Substance Abusers

Mentally ill patients and substance abusers over age 40 years have well-established diseases. Their problems are unique: compliance is universally inadequate; partner cooperation is always a problem; motivation subserves the illness; and high efficacy is required. In addition, medical care is sporadic, resupply rarely occurs regularly, and the medical profession may be indifferent. Vaginal bleeding may often intervene and sexual activity, which is usually intermittent, often results in sexually transmitted diseases. Medical treatment of mental illness often leads to amenorrhea and confusion about the actual need for contraception. Oral contraceptives may be optimal for institutionalized or closely monitored women. Progestin implants, DMPA, or monthly injectable contraceptives may be helpful for the noncompliant. Condoms are essential to prevent STDs, and IUDs do not. Sterilization consent is most difficult to obtain [47].

H. Gynecological Disorders

An intrauterine device is a reasonable option among women with gynecologic problems, which are often prevalent after age 40 years. Uterine leiomyomata that do not distort the endometrial cavity will not decrease the effectiveness of the intrauterine device. However, when distortion exists, it may not be possible to place the IUD at the fundus and diffusion of the copper ion throughout the endometrial cavity may be impaired, inhibiting the contraceptive effectiveness.

Menorrhagia, or irregular menses (once cancer has been ruled out), may benefit from progesterone-containing IUDs.

Uterine or cervical cancer, or genital bleeding of unknown cause, is an absolute contraindication to IUD insertion. Acute cervicitis or actinomycosis must be resolved prior to insertion. An IUD is not recommended if a woman or her partner has multiple sex partners, or may have increased susceptibility to infection (leukemia, AIDS).

I. Interaction of OC's With Other Medications

The concerns of interaction of hormonal contraceptives with other medications are not so much of an adverse reaction, but more that of the other medications affecting the metabolism or bioavailability of the OCs and the OC's effect on the concomitant medication. Traditionally, most of the attention has been focused on the efficacy of OCs, because most women taking OCs are young and take no additional medication

Table 5 The Effects of Antibiotics on the Metabolism of Contraceptive Pills

Antibiotic	Estrogen (μm)	Progestin (mg)	Antibiotic	Steroids
Tetracycline 500 mg qid × 1–5 days	EE 0.35	NE 1.0 mg	0	0
Ciprofloxacin 500 mg bid × 7 days	EE 0.02	Gest 0.075 Levo 0.05–0.15	N/a	0
Ampicillin 500 mg bid 1–5 days	EE 0.030	NE 1.0	0	0
Metronidazole 400 mg tid 6–8 days	EE 0.030	NE 1.0	0	0
Temofloxin 600 mg bid × 7 days	EE 0.030	Levo 0.150	0	0
Doxycycline 100 mg bid × 7 days	EE 0.035	NE 1.0	N/a	0
Rifampin 400–600 mg/ days	—	NE 1.0	N/a	AUC + $t_{1/2}$ reduced

EE = ethiryl estradiol; Gest = gestadene; Levo = levonorgestrel; NE = norethindrone; 0 = no effect; N/a = not assayed.
Pharmacokinetics: AUC/$t_{1/2}$ (red) = area under curve and $t_{1/2}$ of disappearance from the blood reduced.
Sources: Refs. 47–52.

other than an occasional antibiotic for a brief acute infection. Fortunately, nonsteroidal anti-inflammatory drugs (NSAIDS) have no effects on liver metabolism of OC, because NSAIDS primarily excreted through the kidney, and thus have no effect on OC efficacy.

As shown in Table 5 [48–53], antibiotics (except rifampin) have little influence on OC efficacy. However, as women age, incidence increases of other disease's, for which many take additional medication.

Thyroid Disease

Hypothyroidism is common among women, and the incidence increases with age. Acquired impairment of thyroid function in adult women is about 2% in North America [54]. Menopausal hypothyroid women receiving estrogen replacement may have a significant increase in thyroxine—binding globulin and serum total thyroxine levels accompanied by a significant decrease in free thyroxine concentration [55]. This altered thyroid binding may result in a need for more thyroxine to achieve the same therapeutic effect.

IX. CONCLUSION

Contraception in women older than 40 years is different only in that practitioners must consider the concomitant disease and medications of the older woman, plus the well-understood reality that sterilization is an appropriate and popular recommendation. Barrier contraception must be borne in mind, particularly in the face of STDs for the older woman.

REFERENCES

1. U.S. Bureau of the Census, Statistical abstract of the United States 1999 (199th edition), Washington, DC, 1999; Section 2. Vital Statistics, 78.
2. Glasier A, Gebbie A. Contraception for the older woman. Ballière's Best Pract Res Clin Obstet Gynaecol 1996; 10:121-138.
3. U.S. Bureau of the Census, Statistical abstract of the United States 1999 (199th edition), Washington, DC, 1999; Section 2. Vital Statistics, 76.
4. Reid RL. Which contraceptive methods are suitable for the older woman. J Soc Obstet Gynaecol Can 1993; 15:933–944.

5. U.S. Bureau of the Census, Statistical abstract of the United States 1999, Washington, DC, 1999; Section 2. Vital Statistics, 91.

6. Menken J, Trussell J, Larsen U. Age and infertility. Science 1986; 233: 1389–1394.

7. U.S. Bureau of the Census, Statistical abstract of the United States 1999, Washington, DC, 1999; Section 2. Vital Statistics, 89.

8. Hankinson SE, Hunter DJ, Dolditz GA, Willett WC, Stampfer MJ, Rosner B, Hennekens CH, Speizer FE. Tubal ligation, hysterectomy and risk of ovarian cancer. A prospective study. JAMA 1993; 270:2813–2818.

9. Sidney S, Petitti DB, Quesenberry CP Jr, Klatsky AL, Ziel HK, Wolf S. Myocardial infarction in users of low-dose oral contraceptives Obstet Gynecol 1996; 88:934–944.

10. Thomas DB. The WHO Collaborative Study of neoplasia and steroid contraceptives: the influence of combined contraceptives on risk of neoplasms in developing and developed countries. Contraception 1991; 43: 695–710.

11. Herbst AL, Berek JS. Impact of contraception on gynecological cancers. Am J Obstet Gynecol 1993; 168:1980–1985.

12. Poulter NR, Chang CL, Farley TMM, Kelaghan J, Meirlk O, Marmot MG. World Health Organization Collaborative Study of cardiovascular disease and steroid hormone contraception: acute myocardial infarction and combined oral contraceptives: results of an international multicentre case-control study. Lancet 1997: 349:1202–1209.

13. Pettiti DB, Sidney S, Bernstein A, Wolf S, Quesenberry C, Ziel HK. Stroke in users of low-dose contraceptives. N Engl J Med 1996; 335: 8–15.

14. Lidegaard O. Oral contraception and risk of a cerebral thrombo-embolic attack: results of a case-control study. Br Med J 1993; 306:956–963.

15. Suissa S, Blais L, Spitzer WO, Cusson J, Lewis M, Heinemann L. First time use of newer oral contraceptives and the risk of venus thromboembolism. Contraception 1997; 56:141–146.

16. Lewis MA, Heinemann LAJ, Spitzer WO, MacRae KD, Bruppacher R. For the transnational study on oral contraceptives and the health of young women: The use of oral contraception and the occurrence of acute myocardial infarction in young women. Contraception 1997; 56:129–140.

17. Harrison PF, Rosenfield A. Research, introduction, and use: advancing from Norplant. Contraception 1998; 58:323–334.

18. Shangold G, Fisher AC, Rubin A. Pharmacodynamics of the contraceptive patch. Obstet Gynecol 2000; 95 (4 suppl 1):36S.
19. Creasy G, Hall N, Shangold G. Patient adherence with the contraceptive patch dosing schedule versus oral contraceptives. Obstet Gynecol 2000; 95(suppl 1):60S.
20. Hall PE. New once-a-month injectable contraceptives, with particular reference to Cycloefem/Cyclo-Provera. Int J Gynaecol Obstet 1998; 62(Suppl 1):S43.
21. Said S, Sadek W, Kholeif A. For a multi-centered phase III comparative study of two hormonal contraceptive preparations given once-a-month by intramuscular injection: II. The comparison of bleeding patterns. Contraception 1989; 40:531–551.
22. Bahamondes L, Lavin P, Ojeda G, Petta C, Diaz J, Maradiegue E, Monteiro I. Return of fertility after discontinuation of the once-a month injectable contraceptive Cyclofem. Contraception 1997; 55:307–310.
23. Kaunitz AM, Garceau RJ, Cromie MA. Comparative safety, efficacy, and cycle control of Lunelle® monthly contraceptive injection (medroxyprogesterone acetate and estradiol cypionate injectable suspension) and Ortho-novum 7/7/7 oral contraceptives (norethindrone/ethinyl estradiol triphasic). Lunelle® Study Group. Contraception 1999; 60:179–187.
24. Schwallie PC, Assenzo JR. The effect of depo-medroxyprogesterone acetate on pituitary and ovarian function and the return of fertility after its discontinuation; a review. Contraception 1974; 9:181–202.
25. Sulak PJ. Intrauterine device practice guidelines: patient types. Contraception, 1998; 58(suppl 3):55S–58S.
26. Hannaford PC, Kay CR. Oral contraceptives and diabetes mellitus. Br Med J 1989; 299:1315–1316.
27. Garg SK, Chase HP, Marshall G, Hoops SL, Holmes DL, Jackson WE. Oral contraceptives and renal and retinal complications in young women with insulin-dependent diabetes mellitus. JAMA 1994; 271:1099–1102.
28. Klein BEK, Moss SE, Klein R. Oral contraceptives in women with diabetes. Diabetes Care 1990; 13:895–898.
29. Konje JC, Otolorin EO, Ladipo OA. The effect of continuous subdermal levonorgestrel (Norplant) on carbohydrate metabolism. Am J Obstet Gynecol 1992; 166:15–19.
30. Kjos SL, Peters RK, Xiang A, Thomas D, Schaefer U, Buchanan TA. Contraception and the risk of type 2 diabetes mellitus in Latina women with prior gestational diabetes mellitus. JAMA 1998; 280:533–538.
31. Kimmerle R, Berger M, Weiss R, Kurz K. Effectiveness, safety, and

acceptability of a copper intrauterine device (CU Safe 300) in type I diabetic women. Diabetes Care 1993; 16:1227–1230.

32. Skouby SO, Molsted-Pedersen L, Kosonen A. Consequences of intrauterine contraception in diabetic women. Fertil Steril 1984; 42:568–572.

33. Knopp RH, La Rosa JC, Burkman RT. Contraception and dyslipidemia. Am J Obstet Gynecol 1993; 168:1994–2005.

34. Stampfer MJ, Hu FB, Anson JAE, Rimm EB, Willett WC. Primary prevention of coronary heart disease through diet and lifestyle. N Engl J Med 2000; 343:16–22.

35. Narkiewiaz K, Granierto GR, D'este D, Mattarai M, Zonzin P, Palatin P. Ambulatory blood pressure in mild hypertensive women taking oral contraceptives. A case-controlled study. Am J Hypertens 1995; 8:249–253.

36. DeCherney A. Bone-sparing properties of oral contraceptives. Am J Obstet Gynecol 1996; 174:15–20.

37. De Abood M, de Castillo Z, Guerrero F, Espino M, Austin KL. The effect of Depo-Provera or Microgynon on the painful crises of sickle cell anemia patients. Contraception 1997; 56:313–316.

38. DeCeulaer K, Gruber C, Hayes R, Serjeant GR. Medroxyprogesterone acetate and homozygous sickle cell disease. Lancet 1982; 2:229–231.

39. O'Meara ES, Rossing MA, Daling JR, Elmore JG, Barlow WE, Weiss NS. Hormone replacement therapy after a diagnosis of breast cancer in relation to recurrence and mortality. J Natl Cancer Inst 2001; 93:754–762.

40. Mattson RH, Rebar RW. Contraceptive methods for women with neurologic disorders. Am J Obstet Gynecol 1993; 168:2027–2032.

41. Chang CL, Donaghy M, Poulter N. Migraine and stroke in young women: case control study. The World Health Organisation Collaborative Study of Cardiovascular Disease and Steroid Hormone Contraception. Br Med J 1999; 318:13–18

42. Mattson RH, Cramer JA, Caldwell BV, Siconalfi BC. Treatment of seizures with medroxyprogesterone acetate: preliminary report. Neurology 1984; 34:1255–1258.

43. Mattson RH, Cramer JA, Darney PD, Naftolin F. Use of oral contraceptives by women with epilepsy. JAMA 1986; 256:238–240.

44. ACOG Practice bulletin. The use of hormonal contraception in women with coexisting medical conditions. Clinical Management Guidelines for Obstetrician-Gynecologists. 2000; 18:1071–1084.

45. Tang MX, Jacobs D, Stern Y. Effect of oestrogen during menopause on risk and age onset of Alzheimer's disease. Lancet 1996; 348:439–442.

46. Yaffe K, Krueger K, Sarkar S, Grady D, Barrett-Connor E, Cox DA, Nickelsen T, for the multiple outcome of raloxifene investigators. Cognitive function in postmenopausal women treated with raloxifene. N Engl J Med 2001; 344:1207–1213.

47. Hankoff LD, Darney PD. Contraceptive choices for behaviorally disordered women Am J Obstet Gynecol 1993; 1681:1986–1989.

48. Back DJ, Breckenridge AM, Crawford F, MacIver M, Orme ML, Park BK, Rowe PH, Smith E. The effect of rifampicin on norethisterone pharmacokinetics. Eur J Clin Pharmacol 1979; 15:193–197.

49. Neely JL, Abate M, Swinker M, D'Angio R. The effect of doxycycline on serum levels of ethinyl estradiol, norethisterone and endogenous progesterone. Obstet Gynecol 1991; 77:416–420.

50. Back DJ, Tjia J, Martin C, Millar E, Maut T, Morrison P, Orme M. The lack of interaction between temafloxacin and combined oral contraceptives. Contraception 1991; 43:317–323.

51. Joshi JV, Joshi UM, Sankholi GM, Krishna U, Mandlekar A, Chowdury V, Hazari K, Gupta K, Sheth UK, Saxena BN. A study of the interaction of low-dose combination oral contraceptive with ampicillin and metronidazole. Contraception 1980; 22:641–652.

52. Murphy AA, Zacur HA, Charache P, Burkman RT. The effect of tetracycline on levels of oral contraceptives. Am J Obstet Gynecol 1991; 164: 26–33.

53. Maggiolo F, Puricelli G, Dottorini M, Caprioli S, Bianchi W, Suter F. The effect of ciprofloxin on oral contraceptive treatments. Drugs Exp Clin Res 1991; 17:451–454.

54. Wilson JD, Foster DW, Kronenberg HM, Larsen PR, eds. Williams Textbook of Endocrinology. 9th ed. Philadelphia: WB Saunders, 1998: 460.

55. Arafah BM. Increased need for thyroxine in women with hypothyroidism during estrogen therapy. N Engl J Med 2001; 344:1743–1749.

2

Ultralow-Dose Oral Contraception

Sally E. Perlman
The University of Louisville School of Medicine,
Louisville, Kentucky, U.S.A.

Joseph S. Sanfilippo
The University of Pittsburgh School of Medicine and Magee-
Women's Hospital, Pittsburgh, Pennsylvania, U.S.A.

If one were to turn the time clock back to the 1960s, it would become noteworthy that oral contraceptives became available as one prescribed method of contraception. The initial preparation was a "high-dose" formulation. Specifically, a 150-µg estrogen preparation of mestranol was combined with approximately 10 mg of the progestin norethynodrel. The mechanism of action was predicated on inhibition of ovulation. As time progressed, it became evident that lower doses of hormone were just as effective and had fewer untoward effects. Since 1988, no oral contraceptive has been produced with more than 50 µg of ethinyl estradiol or biological equivalent amounts of other estrogens [1]. In 1992 in the United States, a 35-µg preparation was introduced [2]. Ethinyl estradiol and mestranol were the two estrogens used. With the advent of lower-dose estrogen pills, simultaneously a number of progestational preparations became available. Synthetic preparations included norethindrone, norethindrone acetate, levonorgestrel, norgestrel, as well as ethynodiol diacetate and norethynodel. The clinician was able to prescribe oral contraceptives (OCs) designed to meet the hormonal needs of the patient by varying the estrogen, progesterone, and androgen characteristics. Newer progestins with less androgenic activity

23

were subsequently released and include gestodene (GSD), norgestimate, and desogestrel (DSG). The latter preparations are often termed
"third generation" progestins. More recently, a new progestogen with
drospirenone has been introduced, with even more reported antiandro-
genic and antimineralocorticoid effects [3].

As a distinct effort is made to identify the lowest dose, most effective oral contraceptive, 15- to 25-µg preparations of ethinyl estradiol
are currently being evaluated. Currently, all of the newer oral contraceptives being introduced have only one estrogen: ethinyl estradiol.
Variations occur in the type of progestin and in the different dosing
patterns of both estrogen and progestin. Side effects of oral contraceptive preparations have been ascribed to both estrogen and progestin
components. Hence, dosage reductions are indicated in an effort to minimize side effects.

I. MECHANISM OF ACTION OF ORAL
CONTRACEPTIVES

Oral contraceptives inhibit ovulation with the constant level of estrogen
suppressing pituitary gonadotropins [4]. In addition, cervical mucus
changes adversely affecting sperm penetration, decreased tubal motility, and atrophic endometrium are a reflection of progestin component.

The ultralow dose OC began to clinically emerge in the 1990s.
To date, there are approximately seven OC formulations available in
the United States and internationally. They all have ethinyl estradiol.
The dosing is 15, 20, and 25 µg in the monophasic brands and 20,
30, and 35 µg in the triphasic brands. The progestin content includes
primarily 150 µg of DSG or 75 µg of GSD, with one brand each using
1 µg of norethindrone [5] or 100 µg of levonorgestrel [6]. Currently,
there is one type of triphasic progestin scheme. This uses 100-µg DSG
days 1–7, 125-µg DSG days 8–14, and 150-µg DSG days 15–21 [7].

These pills continue to be based on the mechanism of suppression
of ovulation. Although the majority are designed as the higher estrogen-
dosed OCs to be taken for 21 days with 7 days of placebo, two types
have addressed the hormonal changes that occur in the placebo period.
With this low estrogen dosing in some of the 20-µg ethinyl estradiol

OCs with either 150-µg of DSG or 75-µg of GSD, ovulation seemed suppressed, but follicular development and circulating Estradiol (E_2) levels are greater than those with 30-µg ethinyl estradiol preparations [8].

Three groups have studied the effects of circulating hormones and follicular development by decreasing the pill-free interval. One type of OC has 20-µg of ethinyl estradiol and has reduced the pill-free interval to 2 days followed by 5 days of 10 µg of ethinyl estradiol [9]. Two other ultralow-dose OC's have reduced the placebo to 5 days. One used 20 µg of ethinyl estradiol, and the other used 15 µg of ethinyl estradiol [8]. The 20-µg preparations have found reduced ovarian activity. The 15-µg preparation of ethinyl estradiol has found greater variation in the interval between cessation of active treatment and ovulation. The mean estradiol level each day is lower. The authors have postulated that this could represent breakthrough ovulation [8].

II. FAILURE RATES

It has become increasingly obvious that oral contraceptives are highly effective in preventing pregnancy. Overall failure rates are interpreted in terms of women-years (of use). This is termed the Pearl index. Appropriate use of oral contraceptive therapy results in failure rates of less than 1 : 100 women-years when compliance accommodated vs. data attesting to pregnancy rates of 15 : 100 women-years among inner-city teenagers [2].

Despite the concerns about breakthrough ovulation the Pearl index for the ultralow-dose OC remains low. The Pearl index has ranged from 0 to 2.0, compared to matched controls taking 30–35 µg of ethinyl estradiol preparations with a Pearl index of 0–1.2 [10].

III. BENEFITS OF ORAL CONTRACEPTIVE THERAPY

In one sense oral contraceptives can improve "quality of life." If one considers a lower incidence of dysmenorrhea, benign breast disease, iron-deficiency anemia, menstrual irregularities (including dysfunctional uterine bleeding), as well as improvement of acne occurs, then it is logical to consider prescribing for noncontraceptive indications. Table 1 identifies the noncontraceptive benefits of oral contraceptives.

Dysfunctional uterine bleeding is a persistent problem. Davis has reported there is overall improvement in dysfunctional uterine bleeding with ethinyl estradiol- and norgestimate-containing preparations [11].

With few studies to date, the data for the ultralow-dose OC are limited. They have all looked at bleeding patterns and compared them to higher-dose preparations. In general, the ultralow-dose preparations have had patterns consistent with higher doses. The intermenstrual bleeding occurs more often in the first three to four cycles and decreases with longer duration of use. An interest in the progestin role contributing to this pattern has emerged from these studies' variation primarily of the progestin [10]. To date it seems from one study that norethindrone acetate has the least favorable bleeding profile [10]. Most studies showed a consistent 2% withdrawal rate due to bleeding.

Table 1 Noncontraceptive Benefits of Oral Contraceptives

Menstrual improvements
    More regular and predictable menses
    Reduced prevalence and severity of dysmenorrhea
    Reduction in days and amount of menstrual flow
    Increased iron stores in women with menorrhagia
    Restoration of regular menses in anovulatory women
Prevention of benign conditions
    Benign breast disease (fibroadenoma and cystic changes)
    Pelvic inflammatory disease
    Ectopic pregnancy
Prevention of gynecological malignancies
    Epithelial ovarian cancer
    Endometrial adenocarcinoma
Possible benefits
    Prevention of functional ovarian cysts
    Prevention of rheumatoid arthritis
    Increased bone mineral density

Source: Ref. 2.

Primary dysmenorrhea oftentimes improves with OCs. Inhibition of ovulation appears to be the primary explanation for improvement in dysmenorrhea [12,13]. Several studies have shown no difference when the ultralow-dose OC compared with a 30- to 35-μg preparation in the treatment of dysmenorrhea [14].

Oral contraceptives have also been associated with a lower incidence of pelvic inflammatory disease (PID); however, reports are conflicting. Cervical ectopy is an independent risk factor for contraceptive cervicitis, in part due to the columnar cells of the cervix being more susceptible. Several studies have reported reduced rates of chlamydial PID, gonococcal PID, and PID unspecified among users of an OC [1]. Several mechanisms could explain this protective effect. One effect may be from progestins changing cervical and tubal mucous. Another mechanism may be decreased menstrual flow. Despite these studies, the topic remains controversial. Some critics state that most of these studies have used patients with symptomatic disease. Hence, there may be milder cases in which the OC does not protect against the long-term pelvic scarring of asymptomatic PID [1].

A 40% reduction in the risk of ovarian malignancy as well as borderline epithelial ovarian cancer has been reported [14]. Of interest, the effect seems to occur within several cycles of initiation of oral contraceptive therapy and appears to last for 10–15 years after discontinuance [15]. The lowest effective dose to accomplish this has not been clearly defined; although, 35-μg preparations have been noted to have a lower incidence of ovarian cancer [16].

In addition, a 50% risk reduction with respect to endometrial adenocarcinoma has been reported [17]. This effect seems to persist for up to 15 years following discontinuation of an OC [18].

There are no conclusions to date on the effects of ultralow-dose OCs on gynecological and other cancers. In addition, there is no information on benign gynecological conditions, such as PID, fibrocystic breast disease, and ovarian cysts.

Clinicians must be cognizant of research related to OCs and bone mineral density. In light of the pharmacological dose of estrogen, oral contraceptives have a positive effect on bone mineral density [19]. They prevent acceleration of bone turnover and reversal of decreasing bone density in the menopausal female [20]. Two studies with small patient numbers show that the 20-µg ethinyl estradiol OC prevents bone turnover in perimenopausal women [10].

IV. POTENTIAL ADVERSE EFFECTS OF ORAL CONTRACEPTIVES

A. Thromboembolic Disease

Common fears of thromboembolic disease and cancer have repeatedly surfaced. With respect to thromboembolism, individuals taking OC appear to demonstrate a relationship between the dose of the estrogen component and the incidence of thromboembolic phenomena. Low-dose OCs (<35 µg) are associated with less risk of thromboembolism than the earlier preparations [2,21,22]. Controversy within the literature still exists comparing hemorrhagic and ischemic stroke among low-dose OC users with the norgestrel-type progestins. There was an increased risk in the Schwartz et al. Study in Washington state as opposed to the Kaiser Permanente study in Northern and Southern California [22]. Review of U.S. and European studies showed a difference between use of low-dose oral contraceptive and thromboembolic conditions affecting arterial system, ischemic stroke, and myocardial infarction. U.S. studies showed no risk. European studies showed no difference between oral contraceptive generations with respect to accuracy incidence of ischemic stroke. However, risk of myocardial infarction associated with oral contraceptive use consistently was lower for third-generation than second-generation pills [23].

Women in the perimenopausal age range who are particularly concerned about the potential for pregnancy would clearly be another population that could theoretically benefit from low-dose OCs. To date, there are evidence-based studies identifying no increased risk of myocardial infarction or stroke among healthy nonsmoking women who are over 35 years of age and are taking OCs of <50 µg [20,22,24].

The epidemiological studies regarding smoking and oral contraceptives in women over the age of 35 years have addressed the question of risk of arterial events with >50-µg OC preparations. In a case-controlled study, there was no evidence that the use of <50-µg preparations was associated with any increased risk of myocardial infarction or stroke [22,24]. However, smoking continues to be the single most important preventable cause of death and disability in the United States [25]. The number of cigarettes smoked per day is critical and most definitions of "smokers" include those who smoke >15 cigarettes per day.

The problem of hypertension and OCs is of interest. Oral contraceptives appear to increase blood pressure, including the 30-μg ethinyl estradiol preparations. A study conducted by Cardoso et al. assessed 30 μg of ethinyl estradiol and 150 μg of progestin, for which an increase in blood pressure of normotensive women occurred at the level of 8 mm Hg systolic and 6 mm Hg diastolic. If the patient had established hypertension an additional 7 mm Hg blood pressure increase resulted [26,27].

In the Schwartz pooled analysis of two U.S. studies of young users of the low-dose oral contraceptive, very few users were cigarette smokers and/or treated for hypertension. Given the limited data power, one should use the low-dose OC with caution [22].

Available evidence suggests that for most women who use OCs, there is no greater risk of weight gain than for other sexually active women. Recent clinical trials demonstrate that the 20-μg ethinyl estradiol OCs are not associated with clinically relevant weight gain [6,10]. However, most studies appear not to have a consensus on what constitutes excessive weight gain. Bias may exist if women with large weight gain did not follow up. There needs to be prospective randomized studies assessing weight gain in women using OCs and barrier methods over at least 1 year [28].

In younger populations, concern has been expressed with respect to OCs' effect on height. The evidence-based medicine does not support an adverse effect on height in adolescents that use OCs [29]. Essentially, once an adolescent reaches menarche, the endogenous estrogen production has initiated an epiphyseal closure and this process is not affected by exogenous estrogens, i.e. OC therapy. One must assume that with decreased estrogen the ultralow-dose OC would have the same effect.

One would theorize that decreasing the estrogen component even further would decrease fears of thromboembolic (VTE) disease. In terms of VTE, the studies from the ultralow-dose OC are comparable, but again conclusions may be premature. In the literature to date, in one study a 25-year-old smoker had a myocardial infarction while taking 100-µg levonorgestrel and 20-µg ethinyl estradiol OC [6].

Another study showed one patient taking the 150-µg desogestrel/20-µg ethinyl estradiol OC developed severe hypertension [30]. In that same study, another patient had a thromboembolic event while taking 75-µg gestodene/20-µg ethinyl estradiol, but did smoke and have a family history [30]. The latter study was from a European population. In previous reports, the European studies have higher rates of VTE than U.S. studies. Overall, these are three isolated cases among thousands of cycles, which in general, showed no changes in blood pressure, weight, or other adverse VTE signs. More long-term data are needed. At present there is an ongoing large comparison trial conducted by the Oral Contraceptive and Hemostasis Study Group to further explore the effects of different estrogen doses on hemostatic variables [10].

B. Cancer

With respect to cervical cancer, the controversy continues [17]. The problem with studies to date is the existing confounding factors such as smoking, earlier age at coitarche, and multiple sexual partners, which might predispose the individual to cervical cancer. It has been concluded that if OCs are at all associated with increased risk of cervical neoplasm, the association is of "small magnitude" [2]. The studies with the ultralow-dose OC are too short-term to examine cervical cancer effects.

With respect to breast cancer, the overall incidence does not appear to be increased. However, several studies implicate an increased risk of breast cancer with recent or current OC use. Specifically, detection bias may explain the findings [31]. Overall in the 20–54-year age categories, breast cancer and OC data conclusions state that the overall risk of breast cancer is no different for women who have used OC preparations than those who have not [31]. In addition, an individual who uses the OC with a history of benign breast disease as well as a positive family history of breast cancer does not appear to have an associated increased risk of breast cancer [16].

Women who have taken oral contraceptives and then discontinued them for 10 years or more had no increased risk of breast cancer compared to nonusers. A small but significant increased relative risk (RR) with current users has been reported when compared to those who had utilized but discontinued OC therapy 1–4 years prior (RR 1.24 and RR 1.16, respectively). Furthermore, prior oral contraception users who were surveyed 5–9 years after discontinuing OCs had a RR of 1.07. The increased risk was identified in women with localized disease and there was an associated lower incidence of metastatic disease, which may be a reflection of earlier diagnosis, i.e., women taking OCs are more likely to have regular gynecological examinations [32].

The studies with the ultralow-dose OC to date are too short term and too limited to draw any conclusions regarding breast cancer effects.

C. Effect on Lipids

Most data to date focus on 50- and 35-μg preparations with regard to the effects on the lipid profile. However, the National Cholesterol Education Program has recommended that women with controlled dyslipidemia can be prescribed 35 μg or lower estrogen-containing oral contraceptives. If there is elevated low-density lipoprotein (LDL) cholesterol (>160 mg/dl) or additional risk factors for coronary artery disease, including smoking, diabetes, obesity, hypertension, family history of premature coronary artery disease, high-density lipoprotein (HDL) level <35 mg/dl or triglyceride levels >250 mg/dl, use of alternative contraception is recommended [33].

Studies again are limited both in numbers and length of study period with the ultralow-dose OC. One study of OC use in perimenopausal women consisted of 20-μg ethinyl estradiol/150-μg DSG. It showed total serum cholesterol decreased, HDL cholesterol increased, and no change occurred in triglycerides [20].

Another study in reproductive-age women showed an increase in HDL cholesterol of 3% when a 20-μg ethinyl estradiol was used instead of a similar 30-μg ethinyl estradiol preparation, which resulted in a 9% decrease [10]. When a 20-μg ethinyl estradiol was compared to a 30-μg ethinyl estradiol with DSG, there was an improved LDL cholesterol level [10].

A smaller increase in cholesterol was also observed with a 20-μg ethinyl estradiol OC containing levonorgestrel compared with a 35-μg OC containing norethindrone. In another study, a 20-μg ethinyl estradiol/norethindrone OC had a less beneficial effect on high-density lipoproteins than a 35-μg OC with norgestimate [10].

The remaining studies found no real differences both in lipid levels when 20-μg ethinyl estradiol OCs were compared with higher estrogen doses or different progestins [10].

D. Diabetes Mellitus

In a study involving 43 women with type I diabetes mellitus who were taking oral contraceptives for a mean duration of 3.4 years, when compared to women with type I diabetes who were not using oral contraceptive therapies, the hemoglobin A_1C values were not statistically different between the users and nonusers. The authors conclude that 35-μg OC preparations did not have an adverse effect on diabetes [34]. It does not appear that oral contraceptives are a precipitating factor for development of diabetes [35]. Individuals with gestational diabetes who were followed for up to 7 years postpartum and used oral contraceptives did not have an increased incidence of type II diabetes. Currently, there are no data assessing individuals with more profound degrees of diabetes who also take OCs.

Routine glucose monitoring found no difference when ultralow-dose OCs were compared with OCs of higher dosing [7,9]. However, to date, no specific study has addressed the effect of the ultralow-dose contraceptive on diabetes mellitus.

E. Migraine Headaches

Women with a history of migraine headaches using <50 μg of OC preparation have a clear increase (six-fold risk) of ischemic stroke when compared to women not taking OCs. Smokers without a prior history of migraine headaches, when placed on oral contraceptive therapies, had a 34-fold increased risk of ischemic stroke in association with the development of migraine headaches when taking OCs [36]. On the other hand, Schwartz et al., in a pooled study of patients from

Kaiser in northern and southern California and three Washington state counties, stated that ischemic stroke patients, and to a lesser extent hemorrhagic stroke patients, are more likely to report a history of migraines when compared with controls [22]. These studies are limited by self-reports, inconsistent definitions, and limited statistical power.

Headaches as a subjective complaint were present in women taking ultralow-dose OCs. At present, it does not seem as if headaches exist any more frequently than with higher-dose preparations. Again, the data are limited. There is only one case reported in the literature to date of a migraine headache associated with ultralow-dose OC use. This was a European study with a 20-μg ethinyl estradiol/75-μg GSD preparation [29]. One patient reported two episodes of a migraine-like headache.

F.   Seizure Disorders

Specific medications that enhance hepatic enzyme activity include phenobarbital, phenytoin, carbamazepine, felbamate, and topiramate [25]. It has been shown that the efficacy of such anticonvulsant medications is decreased with traditional ($>35\mu g$) oral contraceptive preparations. In addition, the contraceptive efficacy may be decreased as well. Theoretical considerations for the ultralow-dose OCs might include individuals who are taking anticonvulsants that induce hepatic enzyme activity. Given the lower dose of estrogen, it is possible that there is not as much competition with the hepatic enzyme system, and hence the oral contraceptive pill's efficacy may be preserved. Obviously, actual studies need to be done before this medication can be safely used in this population.

Alternative anticonvulsants such as valproic acid, gabapentin, and tiagabine do not appear to decrease levels of contraceptive efficacy while addressing the seizure disorders. This information should be considered by clinicians addressing patients with seizure disorders [25].

G.   Sickle Cell Disease

Sickle cell disease, with its associated abnormal hemoglobin, produces vaso-occlusive problems. No well-controlled studies regarding the potential for VTE in OC users with sickle cell disease has been reported. Two control studies have assessed the use of alternatives, such as depot medroxyprogesterone acetate (DMPA) as an effective method of contraception with sickle cell disease [37,38]. No studies to date have used the ultralow-dose OC in sickle cell disease.

H. Leiomyomata

The predominance of information is that uterine fibroids do not seem to undergo significant increase in size when patients are taking low-dose OC pills [25]. Although there are no studies to date, one would assume the same neutral effects with the ultralow-dose OC.

V. POSTPARTUM AND LACTATING WOMEN

Combined oral contraceptives are not the contraceptive of choice for breastfeeding mothers. There is well-proven evidence of a decrease in milk supply, even for those taking low-dose preparations [39]. There is controversy about when to start the oral contraceptive in non-breastfeeding mothers as to whether there is an increased risk of thromboembolic events immediately in the postpartum period [39].

No specific information is currently available about preparations containing 15, 20, and 25 µg of synthetic estrogen with respect to initiation in the postpartum period or during lactation. However, one could theorize that with even less estrogen, there may be a role for these OCs during this period.

VI. CONCLUSIONS

With the current dilemma for healthcare providers of select populations and the decision about whether or not to prescribe OCs, perhaps ultralow-dose pills can fill the void and allow OCs to reach larger patient populations. Specifically, ultra-low dose pills may be especially effective in smokers over 35 years old; individuals with hypertension, diabetes mellitus, migraine headaches, uterine leiomyomata, or lipid disorders; those who are breastfeeding or postpartum; those taking other medical therapy; immediate preoperative candidates; or those with a history of venous thromboembolism, systemic lupus erythematosus (SLE), or sickle cell disease [25].

The studies of the ultralow-dose OCs have been limited to date, with small sample sizes and short durations of study. They have often been limited to a single study of a new preparation. Effects on ovulation suppression and cycle control are very good. Early reports of minimal adverse effects are promising. At present, there are few large, multicenter, randomized prospective studies ongoing. It is hoped that such studies will expand the use of OCs to populations and medical conditions presently contraindicated for their use.

REFERENCES

1. Rosenfeld WD, Swedler JB. Role of hormonal contraception in prevention of pregnancy and sexually transmitted diseases. Adol Med State Art Rev 1992; 3:June.

2. Hormonal Contraception ACOG Technical Bulletin 198, October 1994.

3. Parsey KS, Pong A. An open-label, multicenter study to evaluate Yasmin, a low-dose combination oral contraceptive containing drospirenone, a new progestogen. Contraception 2000; 61:105–111.

4. Letterie GS, Chow GE. Effect of "missed" pills on oral contraceptive effectiveness. Obstet Gynecol 1992; 79:979–982.

5. Rowan JP. Estrophasic dosing: a new concept in oral contraceptive therapy. Am J Obstet Gynecol 1999; 180:3025–3065.

6. Archer D, Maheux R, DelCote A, O'Brien F. North American Levonorgestrel Study Group (NALSG). Efficacy and safety of a low-dose monophasic combination oral contraceptive containing 100 µg levonorgestrel and 20 µg ethinyl estradiol. Am J Obstet Gynecol 1999; 181:539–544.

7. Kaunitz A. Efficacy cycle control and safety of two triphasic oral contraceptives cyllessa™ (Desogestrel/ethinyl estradiol) and Ortho-Novum 7/7/7® (norethindrone/ethynylestradiol). Contraception 2000; 61:295–302.

8. Sullivan H, Furniss H, Spona J, Eisteer M. Effect of 21-day and 24-day oral contraceptive regimens containing gestodene (60 µg) and ethinyl estradiol (15 µg) on ovarian activity. Fertil Steril 1999; 72:115–120.

9. Mircette Study Group. An open label of multicenter non-comparative safety and efficacy study of Mircette, a low dose estrogen–progesterone oral contraceptive. Am J Obstet Gynecol 1998; 179:25-28.

10. Poindexter A. Emerging use of the 20 µg oral contraceptive. Fertil Steril 2001; 75:457–465.

11. Davis, A. Triphasic norgestimate-ethinyl estradiol for treating dysfunctional uterine bleeding. Obstet Gynecol 2000; 96:913–920.

12. VanHooff M, Hirasing R, Kaprin M, Koppenaac C, VoorHorst F, Schoemaker J. The use of oral contraception by adolescents for contraception, menstrual cycle problems or acne. Acta Obstet Gynecol Scand 1998; 77:898–904.

13. Robertson J, Plichţa S, Weisman C, Nathanson C, Ensminger M. Dysmenorrhea and use of oral contraceptives in adolescent women attending a family planning clinic. Am J Obstet Gynecol 1992; 166:578–583.

14. Bassol S, Acvarado A, Celis C, Cravioto M, Perelta O, Montano R, Novelli J, Albornor H, Baiamondes L, Demelo N, Reyes-Marquez R, Acbrecht G. Latin American experience with two low-dose oral contraceptives containing 30 µg ethinyl estradiol 75 µg gestodene and 20 µg ethinyl estradiol 150 µg desogestrel. Contraception 2000; 62:131–135.

15. Hankinson SE, Golditz GA, Hunter DJ, Spencer TL, Rosner B, Stampfer MJ. A quantitative assessment of oral contraceptive use and risk of ovarian cancer. Obstet Gynecol 1992; 80:708–714.

16. The Cancer and Steroid Hormone Study of the Centers for Disease Control and the National Institute of Child Health and Human Development. The reduction in risk of ovarian cancer associated with oral-contraceptive use. N Engl J Med 1987; 316:650–655.

17. Schlesselman JJ. Cancer of the breast and reproductive tract in relation to use of oral contraceptives. Contraception 1989; 40:1–38.

18. The Centers for Disease Control Cancer and Steroid Hormone Study. Oral contraceptive use and the risk of endometrial cancer. JAMA 1983; 249:1600–1604.

19. Gambacciani M, Spinetti A, Taponeco F, Cappagli B, Piaggesi L, Fiorett P. Longitudinal evaluation of perimenopausal vertebral bone loss: effects of a low-dose oral contraceptive preparation on bone mineral density and metabolism. Obstet Gynecol 1994; 83:392–396.

20. Van Winter JT, Bernard M. Oral contraceptive use during the perimenopausal years. Am Fam Physician 1998; 58:1373–1377, 1381-1382.

21. Gertsman BB, Poper JM, Tomita DK, Ferguson WJ, Stadel BV, Lundin FE. Oral contraceptive estrogen dose and the risk of deep venous thromboembolic disease. Am J Epidemiol 1991; 133:32–37.

22. Schwartz SM, Petitti D, Siscovick D, Longstreth WT, Sidney S, Raghunathan T, Wuesenberry C, Kelaghan J. Stroke and use of low-dose oral contraceptives in young women: a pooled analysis of two US studies. Stroke 1998; 29:2277–2284.

23. Lewis MA. Myocardial infarction and stroke in young women: what is the impact of oral contraceptives? Am J Obstet Gynecol 1998;179:S68–S77.

24. Sidney S, Siscovick DS, Petitti DB, Schwartz SM, Quesenberry CP, Psaty BM, Raghunatha T, Kelaghan J, Koepsell T. Myocardial infarction and use of low-dose oral contraceptives: a polled analysis of 2 US studies. Circulation 1998; 98:1058–1063.

25. Smoking and Women's Health. ACOG Practice Bulletin 1997; 2040.

26. Cardoso F, Polonia J, Santos A, Solva-Carvalho J, Ferreira de Almedi J. Low-dose oral contraceptives and 24 hour ambulatory blood pressure. Int J Gyneacol Obstet 1997; 59:237–243.

27. Narkiewicz K, Graniero G, D'Este D, Mattarei M, Zonzin P, Palatini P. Ambulatory blood pressure in mild hypertensive women taking oral contraceptives. A case-control study. Am J Hypertens 1995; 8:249–253.

28. Gupta S. Weight gain on the combined pill—is it real? Hum Reprod Update 2000; 6:427–431.

29. Bolton G. Adolescent contraception: Clin Obstet Gynecol 1981; 24:977-986.

30. Gnorikat J, Dusterberg B, Ruebiga A, Gerlinger C, Strowitzkit T. Comparison of efficacy. Cycle control and tolerability of two low-dose oral contraceptives in a multicenter clinical study. Contraception 1999; 60: 269–274.

31. Breast cancer and hormonal contraceptions: collaborative reanalysis of individual data on 53,297 with breast cancer and 100,239 without breast cancer from 54 epidemiologic studies. Lancet 1996; 347:1713–1727.

32. Breast cancer and hormonal contraceptives: collaborative reanalysis of individual data on 53,297 with breast cancer and 100,239 without breast cancer from 54 epidemiologic studies. Lancet 1996; 347:1713–1727.

33. National Cholesterol Education Program Expert Panel on Detection, Evaluation, and Treatment of High Blood Cholesterol in Adults. Report of the National Cholesterol Education Program Expert Panel on Detection. Evaluation, and Treatment of High Blood Cholesterok in Adults. Arch Intern Med 1988; 148:36–69.

34. Garg S, Chase H, Marshall G, Hoops S, Holmes D, Jackson W. Oral contraceptives and renal and retinal complications in young women with insulin-dependent diabetes mellitus. JAMA 1994; 271:1099–1102.

35. Chasan-Taber L, Willett W, Stampfer M, Hunter D, Colditz G, Spiegel-
     man D, et al. a prospective study of oral contraceptives and NIDDM
     among U.S. women. Diabetes Care 1997; 20:330–335.
36. Chang C, Donaghy M, Poulter N. Migraine and stroke in young women:
     case control study. The World Health Organisation Collaborative Study
     of Cardiovascular Disease and Steroid Hormone Contraception. Br Med
     J 1999; 318:13–18.
37. De Ceulaer K, Gruber C, Hayes R, Serjeant G. Medroxyprogesterone
     acetate and homozygous sickle-cell disease. Lancet 1982; 2:229–231.
38. de Abood M, de Castillo Z, Guerrero F, Espino M, Austin K. Effect of
     Depo-Provera or Microgyn on the painful crises of sickle cell anemia
     patients. Contraception 1997; 56:313–316.
39. Grimes DA, Wallach M, eds. Modern Contraception. Totowa, NJ: Em-
     ron, 1997.

3

Hormone Replacement Therapy and the Role of Androgens

Camille Sylvestre
McGill University and McGill University Health Centre, Montreal, Quebec, Canada

Morrie M. Gelfand
Sir Mortimer B. Davis Jewish General Hospital and McGill University, Montreal, Quebec, Canada

I. INTRODUCTION

Androgens are important hormones that have diverse actions on sexual behavior, affect, cognitive function, and the maintenance of bone density in women. The decline in the production of ovarian and adrenal androgens that commences in the decade preceding menopause may have an impact on women's health. The clinical sequelae of androgen deficiency in menopausal women have only recently been acknowledged, and androgen replacement for those who are symptomatic is becoming an increasingly important therapeutic option.

It has been known that androgen (A) when added to estrogen (E) improves libido since 1950 [1,2]. The information then was anecdotal, and it was not until the mid-1980s that Sherwin and Gelfand demonstrated that the addition of androgen to estrogen in hormone replacement therapy (HRT) improved sexuality, energy, and well-being as well as augmenting libido [3–6]. Today, the quality of life has become a very pertinent issue in the management of women given HRT.

In both males and females, the synthesis of androgens is triggered by hormonal signals from the hypothalamus and the pituitary gland. In women, testosterone (T) is produced by the ovaries, the adrenal glands, and by peripheral conversion of precursor hormones. Testosterone can be aromatized to estradiol, the most potent female estrogen, by the aromatase enzyme complex. Only 1–2% of total circulating T is free and biologically active. The rest is bound by sex hormone binding globulin (SHBG) and albumin. Increasing levels of estradiol increase SHBG and decrease free T levels, exacerbating T deficiency syndromes.

In a recent Canadian survey, 70.8% of the practitioners stated that they add androgen to estrogen for the enhancement of the quality of life. This is a surprising percentage, considering that 10 years ago probably only 5% of the practitioners even knew about estrogen–androgen HRT. The addition of androgen to estrogen HRT raises the issue of risk problems and secondary effects, and these are issues that must be addressed. In a recent review, the authors (7) concluded that the use of androgens in women has no risk consequences as long as they are used judiciously. Judiciously, in most or every case, means the maintenance of androgen levels within normal limits.

In the management of perimenopausal, menopausal, and postmenopausal patients, there are certain parameters which serve as guidelines to HRT. There are the acute symptoms such as vasomotor and atrophic symptoms, and long-term benefits such as the prevention of osteoporosis, cardiovascular diseases, and senile dementia. The quality of life issue, which is both acute and long term, is the most important. The risks involve the incidence of breast cancer, endometrial cancer, and the possible side effects. In this review, we will discuss the roles of estrogen, progestin, and androgen in HRT.

II. EFFECTS ON SEXUALITY

A. Hormonal Activity in Postmenopausal Women

Premenopausal women produce about 300 μg of testosterone daily, whereas postmenopausal women produce about 180 μg, or about 70%

of the testosterone secreted by reproductive age women. Premenopausal women, who have undergone bilateral oophorectomy, have a
reduction in their testosterone level by 50%; the remaining 50% is from
adrenal gland. Therefore, testosterone production still takes place at a
near-normal level in the first year or two after natural menopause, then
declines gradually. This is in contrast to an abrupt and more complete
decrease in surgical menopause.

The hormonal transition of menopause encompasses decreased
levels of estrogen (up to 80% reduction) and testosterone, the latter
being associated with decreased sexual libido, sensitivity, activity, and
response. Additional genitourinary effects associated with menopause
include atrophic changes in the vagina, vulva, urethra, and the bladder
neck.

The effects of estrogen therapy in postmenopausal women in
maintaining vaginal lubrication, decreasing vaginal atrophy, and increasing pelvic blood flow, and the result of alleviating or preventing
dyspareunia is well documented. However, some patients also require
androgen to improve sexual desire or other sexual problems associated
with menopause. The decrease in free testosterone is due to an increase
in SHBG (possibly caused by estrogen replacement therapy [ERT]),
combined with a reduction in pituitary luteinizing hormone (LH) secretion which lessens the stimulus for ovarian testosterone production (8).

B. Androgen Therapy and Sexual Function

In a randomized, crossover study (4), the role of androgens in the maintenance of sexual function in 60 premenopausal, hysterectomized,
oophorectomized women was evaluated. Five aspects of sexual behaviour were monitored daily for 1 month in 3 groups. Women in group
1 received an estrogen–androgen combination as a monthly intramuscular injection (7.5 mg estradiol dienanthate, 1 mg estradiol benzoate,
150 mg testosterone enanthate benzylic acid hydrazone) after the operation. Women in the second group received estrogen only (10 mg estradiol valerate intramuscular every 28 days), and women in the third
group had no treatment. Plasma estradiol and testosterone levels were
measured at baseline and on days 2, 4, 8, 15, 21 and 28 after the injection. Women treated with estrogen–androgen reported significantly

higher rates of sexual desire, arousal, number of fantasies, rates of coitus, and number of orgasms than did patients treated with estrogen alone or untreated. Changes in these sexual behaviors varied directly with plasma testosterone level, but not with plasma estradiol level. These findings imply that androgens may be critical for the maintenance of optimal levels of sexual function in postmenopausal women.

Davis and McCloud (9,10) conducted a prospective, 2-year, single-blind randomized trial of either estradiol implants 50 mg (E) or estradiol 50 mg plus testosterone 50 mg (E + T) three times a month for 2 years in 34 postmenopausal women. In this study, sexuality was measured at baseline and then every 6 months using the Sabbatsberg Self-Rating Scale (SSS). The SSS measures include libido, sexual activity, satisfaction, pleasure, fantasy, orgasm, and relevancy, the latter being a score of the importance of sexuality in a woman's life. Over the 2 years, the E + T group experienced a greater improvement in sexuality than the E group regarding activity, satisfaction, pleasure, orgasm, and relevancy. The effect of treatment approached significance for libido, but did not differ for fantasy in subjects who received E alone.

Sarrel and Dobay (11) assessed sexual function in a double-blind, active-control, parallel-group study of 20 naturally and surgically menopausal women with inadequate responses to current estrogen therapy. After a 2-week washout period, patients were randomly assigned to receive either 1.25 mg esterified estrogens or 1.25 mg esterified estrogens plus 2.5 mg methyltestosterone daily for 8 weeks. Patients who received short-term esterified estrogen plus methyltestosterone therapy demonstrated significant improvements in sexual desire and sensation compared with improvements achieved with previous estrogen therapy.

Shifren and Braunstein (12) evaluated the effects of transdermal testosterone in 75 women who had impaired sexual function after surgically induced menopause. They all received conjugated equine estrogens 0.625 mg per day orally and either placebo, 150 µg of testosterone, or 300 µg of testosterone per day transdermally for 12 weeks. The serum testosterone levels (still in the normal range) correlated with scores for frequency of sexual activity and pleasure–orgasm. At the higher dose of testosterone, the percentages of women who had sexual fantasies, masturbated, or engaged in sexual intercourse at least once a week increased two or three times from the baseline.

The addition of androgen to estrogen hormonal replacement therapy improves sexual function in terms of libido, sensation, arousal, fantasies, and frequency.

III. PSYCHOLOGICAL EFFECTS

A. Mood Symptoms

During the past three decades, the relationship between mood and menopause has been extensively studied. Results from these studies indicate that there is no specific relationship between natural menopause and mood syndromes. It is to be noted that most women do not have a mood or anxiety disorder. Common postmenopausal symptoms seen in clinical practice include depression, mood swings, irritability, and anxiety. It appears that decreased estrogen impacts on central neurotransmitter release, and has a role in mood and behavior changes. In addition, psychosocial factors related to this period in life may also have an impact on mood.

B. Vasomotor Symptoms

The vasomotor symptoms, such as hot flushes and sleep disturbances consequently causing mood disorders, are known to respond to exogenous administration of estrogens; fatigue, memory problems, anxiety, depression, and agoraphobia also appear to respond to treatment with estrogens. The possible effects of androgens on psychological symptoms associated with menopause has been investigated by several authors.

Burger and Hailes (13) evaluated the use of combined estrogen–androgen therapy for the relief of vasomotor symptoms in 17 menopausal women who had previous failures of estrogen therapy (estradiol 40 mg and testosterone 100 mg injections every 3 months). The treatment provided notable, but not statistically significant relief of hot flushes.

Watts and Notelovitz (14) performed a multicenter, double-blind, crossover study that compared the effects of esterified estrogens alone (1.25 mg oral daily) and in combination with methyltestosterone therapy (2.5 mg daily) in 60 surgically menopausal patients. Both regimens significantly reduced the mean hot flush severity score with respect to baseline, the reduction being faster with androgens. This effect was maintained for the 2-year study period.

Simon and Klaiber (15) showed the beneficial effects of methyltestosterone (0.625 mg of oral esterified estrogens plus 1.25 mg methyltestosterone, or 1.25 mg oral esterified estrogens plus 2.5 mg methyltestosterone) compared with estrogen alone in a 3-month, double-blind, placebo-controlled trial in 92 patients. Esterified estrogens plus methyltestosterone provided greater relief of the menopausal somatic symptoms (hot flushes, sweats, vaginal dryness) than did the corresponding esterified estrogens, and the extent of relief was similar to that observed with the higher dose of esterified estrogens alone (10).

C. Sense of Well-Being

It is now recognized that a decline in testosterone production plays a role in the reduction of sense of well-being and energy. In one study (4), the authors concluded that the sense of well-being and energy level were higher in the androgen-treated women when compared to those untreated or treated with estrogen alone.

IV. EFFECTS ON BONE

A. Estradiol, Androgens and the Risk of Fracture

Osteoporosis is an important health issue in our society with an aging population, especially because 75% of the women affected are postmenopausal. In general, there is a direct correlation between age and the incidence of fractures of the vertebrae, proximal femur, and wrist. However, osteoporotic fractures are the end result of a silent process during which there is a continuous decrease in bone mineral density. The skeletal mass increases steadily until a peak between the ages of

20 and 30 years. After a few years of stability, women face a reduction in bone mass as estradiol levels decrease to <60 pg/ml. This reduction may begin before the onset of menopause. Women lose bone at an accelerated rate, with approximately 10–20% of bone mineral density being lost within the first 10 years after the onset of menopause. By the age of 80 years, White women may have lost as much as 50% of their skeletal mass. Surgical menopause is associated with a sudden and complete loss of ovarian androgen and estrogen production, resulting in earlier and more accelerated bone loss.

Estrogen deficiency has been clearly demonstrated to be a major risk factor for the development of osteoporosis, and this is the first reason to prescribe estrogen replacement therapy; however, recent studies have documented that testosterone also plays an important role in women.

Longcope and Baker (16) measured androgens and estradiol levels in postmenopausal women with vertebral crush fractures. Results were compared with a similar population without vertebral crush fractures. Women with vertebral crush fractures were found to have significantly lower metabolic clearance rates of testosterone and estrone, and also a decreased androgen production.

Johansson and Mellstrom (17) reported that there was significant association of women who had undergone a total abdominal hysterectomy with bilateral salpingo-oophorectomy (at a mean of 45.3 years of age) with significantly lower bone mineral density levels at 70 years of age. In contrast, women who had undergone hysterectomy without bilateral oophorectomy showed a higher bone mineral density in the right calcaneus at 70 years of age than did control subjects.

B.   Effects of Estrogens and Androgens on Bone Physiology

Initial studies have shown that androgens have direct bone-sparing and bone-stimulating effects in postmenopausal women. Testosterone in particular has been shown to stimulate bone formation, stimulate osteoclasts to differentiate and proliferate, inhibit bone resorption, and stimulate muscle strength. Some of the protective action of testosterone with respect to bone physiology may occur through its conversion to estrogen by bone aromatase activity (18), but also through specific androgen receptors on bone.

The different effects of estrogens and androgens on bone markers were evaluated by Raisz and Wiita (19) in 28 postmenopausal women in a double-blind study. Patients were randomly assigned to receive either 1.25 mg conjugated equine estrogens or 1.25 mg esterified estrogens plus 2.5 mg methyltestosterone for 9 weeks. Bone physiology was measured by markers of bone resorption (deoxypyridinoline, pyridinoline, and hydroxyproline) and formation (bone-specific alkaline phosphatase, osteocalcin, and C-terminal procollagen peptide).

With respect to resorption markers, the effects of estrogen and estrogen plus methyltestosterone were similar throughout treatment and post-treatment. There were significant increases, however, in bone-specific alkaline phosphatase, a bone formation marker, in patients who received estrogen plus methyltestosterone with respect to values in the estrogen alone group. These results suggest that androgens do not lessen the beneficial effect of estrogen on bone resorption. Although stimulation increases bone formation, the duration of the study was not long enough to determine whether the positive effects of androgen would result in an increase in bone density beyond that achieved with estrogen replacement therapy alone.

C.   Estrogen–Androgen Therapy and Bone Mineral Density

A number of studies have documented the positive effects of androgens on bone mineral density in naturally and surgically postmenopausal women.

Savvas and Studd (20) determined the effect of subcutaneous estradiol and testosterone replacement on bone density of 20 naturally menopausal women who were receiving long-term oral estrogen therapy. Patients were randomized to one of the two treatments for one year. Patients who received the subcutaneous estradiol and testosterone implants had a significant increase with respect to baseline in spinal (5.7%) and femoral neck (5.2%) bone mineral densities. Patients who continued taking oral estrogen therapy had no change in bone mineral density.

Davis and McCloud (10) investigated the effects of estrogen-androgen therapy on bone density in a prospective, 2-year, single-blind trial in 34 menopausal women. Patients were assigned to either estradiol implants (50 mg) or to estradiol (50 mg) plus testosterone (50 mg) implants every 3 months. Both treatment groups had significant increases with respect to baseline values in total body, lumbar vertebral (L1–L4), and hip bone mineral density, but the increase was greater in the estrogen–androgen therapy group.

Watts and Notelovitz (14) measured lumbar spine and hip bone mineral density in 60 surgically menopausal patients during a 2-year period. Patients were randomized either to esterified estrogens (1.25 mg/day) or esterified estrogens (1.25 mg/day) plus methyltestosterone (2.5 mg/day). All patients received 1500 mg of supplemental calcium. Spine mineral density values increased significantly from baseline after 12 months and 24 months of estrogen–androgen therapy. These authors concluded that both treatments prevented loss of bone mineral density of the lumbar spine and hip, and that patients who received estrogen–androgen therapy benefited from significant increases from baseline spinal bone mineral density at 12 and 24 months.

The Estratest Working Group (21) conducted a double-blind, randomized, 2-year study evaluating the effects of estrogen and estrogen–androgen replacement therapy on 291 surgically menopausal women. Patients were randomly assigned to receive conjugated estrogens at 0.625 mg/day, conjugated estrogens at 1.25 mg/day, esterified estrogens at 0.625 mg/day plus methyltestosterone at 1.25 mg/day, or esterified estrogens at 1.25 mg/day plus methyltestosterone at 2.5 mg/day. During the 2-year study period, patients receiving the estrogen–androgen combination showed greater increases from baseline in bone mineral densities of the hip and spine than did the patients receiving conjugated estrogens alone.

Estrogens and androgens diminish bone resorption, and androgens also enhance bone formation. It has also been shown that 2–4 years after women discontinue estrogen–androgen replacement therapy, their bone mass density continues to improve, unlike women taking estrogen replacement therapy, who upon discontinuing it, begin to lose bone mass (22).

There is thus gathering evidence to promote the idea of adding testosterone to the hormone replacement therapy regimen in order to further decrease the incidence of osteoporosis over and above that induced by estrogens alone. The addition of testosterone to estrogen therapy should be considered not only in physiological menopause, but also in nonphysiological loss of ovarian function, such as in hypothalamic–pituitary disease, premature ovarian failure, oophorectomy, and Turner's syndrome.

V. CARDIOVASCULAR EFFECTS

A. Effects on Lipids

One reason physicians choose not to prescribe estrogen–androgen hormonal replacement therapy stems partly from concern that its use may reverse the increased serum concentration of high-density lipoprotein (HDL) cholesterol that is achieved by estrogen replacement therapy alone. This argument fails to take into consideration that estrogen–androgen HRT significantly lowers serum triglycerides levels, in contrast to ERT alone, which elevates them (22).

Watts and Notelevitz (14) compared the efficacy and safety of 1.25 mg/day oral esterified estrogens with the one of 1.25 mg/day oral esterified estrogens plus 2.5 mg/day methyltestosterone in a double-blind, randomized, 2-year, parallel-group study of 60 surgically menopausal women. In the estrogen–androgen group, total cholesterol, HDL cholesterol, and triglycerides levels were all decreased significantly with respect to baseline. There was a slight but statistically insignificant increase in low density lipoprotein (LDL) cholesterol in that same group. Similar results in lipid profiles with estrogen–androgen therapy were reported after a 2-year study conducted by Barrett-Connor (21). In studies involving injectable testosterone (3,4), the authors did not find any changes in the lipid profiles.

B. Effects on Vasodilation

Research into the impact of estrogen—androgen therapy on nonlipid mechanisms of cardiovascular disease is ongoing. Impaired vasodilation is considered an early indicator of endothelial dysfunction, which in turn is a nonlipid mechanism that may contribute to the pathology of coronary vasospasm and myocardial ischemia.

Honoré and Williams (23) compared the short-term effects (15 weeks) of esterified estrogens plus methyltestosterone, esterified estrogens alone, and placebo on coronary artery reactivity in 36 adults female cynomolgus monkeys who underwent oophorectomy. The monkeys were fed an atherogenic diet. The doses used in this study were equivalent to those of women receiving 2.5 mg esterified estrogens plus 5 mg methyltestosterone. The addition of methyltestosterone did not alter the dilatory response of coronary arteries to acetylcholine in monkeys after 12 weeks of treatment.

Recently, Worboys and Kotsopoulos (24) investigated the effects of testosterone implant therapy on arterial reactivity encompassing endothelial-dependent and -independent vasodilation in women using HRT. Endothelial dysfunction can be assessed in vivo with flow-mediated dilation (FMD). Brachial artery FMD has been correlated with coronary endothelial function and cardiovascular risk factors. It deteriorates following menopause and improves with estrogen therapy. B-mode ultrasound measurements of resting brachial artery diameter, following reactive hyperemia (endothelium-dependent FMD), and following glyceryl trinitrate (GTN) (endothelium-independent dilation), were recorded in 33 postmenopausal women stabilized on HRT (>6 months), at baseline, and 6 weeks after a testosterone implant (60 mg), with 15 postmenopausal nonusers of HRT serving as controls. In the brachial artery, baseline resting diameter was similar. In the treated group, testosterone levels increased, associated with a mean 42% increase in FMD. The control group did not change. Glyceryl trinitrate-induced vasodilation increased with testosterone treatment (14.9%). Their preliminary data indicate that parenteral testosterone improves both endothelial-dependent (flow mediated) and endothelium-independent (GTN mediated) brachial artery vasodilation in postmenopausal women using long-term estrogen therapy.

Androgens have also been found lately to play a role in the cardiac syndrome X. This syndrome is described as the triad of angina pectoris, a positive exercise test for myocardial ischemia, and angiographically normal coronary arteries. Although syndrome X does not result in an increased risk of cardiovascular mortality, the symptoms are often troublesome and unresponsive to conventional antianginal therapy. The patients are postmenopausal, and estrogen therapy can alleviate anginal symptoms. Adamson and Webb (25) investigated the effect of esterified estrogens combined with methyltestosterone (Estratest) for 8 weeks on quality of life in 16 postmenopausal women with syndrome X in a randomized, double-blind, cross-over study. The "emotional" score of the Cardiac Health Profile questionnaire was significantly improved after Estratest use compared with placebo. There was no significant treatment effect on exercise parameters, including time to onset of chest pain. The authors have demonstrated a beneficial effect of Estratest on emotional well-being in postmenopausal women with cardiological syndrome X.

VI. EFFECTS ON ENDOMETRIUM AND BREASTS

One has to remember that with the uterus in place, the addition of androgen to estrogen has an effect on the endometrial response to the hormones. It is known that using 0.625 mg of conjugated estrogens daily for 25–30 days results in 30% hyperplasia at the end of 1 year. The addition of medroxyprogesterone acetate (MPA) in a 5-mg dose from days 15–25 of the 30-day cycle eliminates the hyperplasia. Adding the androgen to estrogen regime increases the number of cases with hyperplasia to 42%. Gelfand and Ferenczy (26) have shown that one has to add 10 mg of MPA from day 12 to 25 of each cycle to reduce the hyperplasia to 0 (4), or add 5 mg every day in a continuous manner.

Lovell (27) has investigated the effects of parenteral estrogen–androgen replacement on the incidence of breast cancer. He reviewed nearly 4000 cases of women who had been treated, and found that the incidence of breast cancer was lower in the treated group compared to the population without treatment.

Other studies have examined the role of androgens in breast cancer itself. Poulin and Baker (28) described the inhibitory effect of 5α-dihydrotestosterone (5α-DHT) and its precursor testosterone (T) on the growth of the estrogen-sensitive human breast cancer cell line ZR-75-1. In the absence of estrogens, cell proliferation measured after a 12-

day incubation period was 50–60% inhibited by maximal concentration of 5α-DHT, T, or androstenedione. The antiestrogen LY156758 induced 25–30% inhibition of basal cell growth, its effect being additive to that of 5α-DHT. The antiproliferative effect of androgens was competitively reversed by the antiandrogen hydroxyflutamide, thus indicating an androgen receptor-mediated mechanism. The present data suggest the potential benefits of an androgen–antiestrogen combination in the endocrine management of breast cancer.

Kellokumpu-Lehtinen and Huovinen (29) compared the response to tamoxifen (TAM) versus nandrolone decanoate (NAN) in previously untreated postmenopausal women with advanced breast cancer. In the 67 patients treated with TAM, 15% had complete or partial remission, 42% had stabilized disease, and 43% had progressive disease; in the 60 patients treated with NAN, the results were 17%, 37%, and 47%, respectively. The authors concluded that TAM and NAN were comparable in the treatment of advanced breast cancer.

VII. EFFECTS ON THE BRAIN

Estrogen can stimulate neuronal growth by increasing synaptic density. Estrogen appears to exert its neurologic effects by blocking calcium channels in cell-membrane receptors, where it also alters chloride, potassium, and sodium channels. Progesterone produces the opposite effect, driving calcium into neurons. In the peripheral nervous system, estrogen has been shown to alter the perception of touch through a direct effect on receptors in pacinian corpuscles located in the glabrous skin of the lips and fingertips (30). Estrogen is also an active neuroprotectant and is presently being investigated as a potential therapy against Alzheimer's disease for women (31).

The effects of androgens on the brain are mediated through androgen receptors but also by the aromatization of testosterone to estradiol. Androgen receptors have been identified in the cortex, pituitary, hypothalamus, preoptic region, thalamus, amygdala, and brain stem. Androgen effects in the brain influence sexual behavior, libido, temperature control, sleep control, assertiveness, cognitive function, and learning capacities, including visual–spatial skills and language fluency.

Recently, Hammond and Le (31) studied the role of male hormones in neuroprotection. It had been observed that men in their sixth decade are usually less prone to Alzheimer's disease than women of the same age, but little is known about the neuroprotective role of androgens on the aging central nervous system. They investigated the effect of testosterone, methyltestosterone, and epitestosterone at physiological concentrations on primary cultures of human neurons induced to undergo apoptosis by serum deprivation. As expected, physiological concentrations of 17β-estradiol and transcriptionally inactive 17α-estradiol protect neurons against apoptosis. Similar to 17β-estradiol, physiological concentrations of testosterone are also neuroprotective. The nonaromatizable androgen, miboterone, is also neuroprotective, and the aromatase inhibitor, 4-androsten-4-OL-3,17-dione, does not prevent testosterone-mediated neuroprotection. In contrast, the antiandrogen flutamide eliminates testosterone-mediated neuroprotection. The testosterone analog, methyltestosterone, showed androgen receptor-dependent neuroprotection that was delayed in time, indicating that a metabolite may be the active agent. The endogenous antiandrogen, epitestosterone, also showed a slight neuroprotective effect, but not through the androgen receptor. These results indicate that androgens induce neuroprotection directly through the androgen receptor, and that they may be of therapeutic value against Alzheimer's disease.

VIII.   CONCLUSIONS

1. Postmenopausal ovaries produce androgen.
2. Patients who have undergone bilateral oophorectomy have a particular need for estrogen–androgen hormone replacement therapy, but postmenopausal women with intact ovaries should also be considered as candidates.
3. Estrogen–androgen hormone replacement therapy in patients who have an intact uterus necessitates the addition of MPA 10 mg daily from day 12 to 25 of the cycle.
4. Sexuality in terms of desire, fantasies, and arousal is enhanced by the addition of androgens to the estrogen hormone replacement regimen.

5. Well-being, energy level, and vasomotor symptoms are improved with estrogen–androgen replacement therapy.
6. Estrogen–androgen replacement therapy increases bone mineral density and bone formation above estrogen replacement alone.
7. Long-term estrogen–androgen replacement therapy has not been shown to affect the lipid profile adversely. It also increases the dilation of coronary arteries, when taken parenterally.
8. Androgens have a neuroprotective effect and could be used against Alzheimer's disease.
9. Patients should be given the choice of receiving estrogen–androgen hormone replacement therapy when its need is clinically evident.

REFERENCES

1. Greenblatt RB, Williams E, Barfield. Evaluation of an estrogen-androgen combination and a placebo in the treatment of the menopause. J Clin Endocrinol Metab 1950; 10:1547–1558.
2. Grody MH, Lampie EH. Estrogen-androgen substitution therapy in the aged female. Obstet Gynecol 1953; 2:36–41.
3. Sherwin BB, Gelfand MM. Sex steroids and effect in the surgical menopause: a double-blind, cross-over study. Psychoneuroendocrinology 1985; 10:325–335.
4. Sherwin BB, Gelfand MM. The role of androgen in the maintenance of sexual functioning in oophorectomized women. Psychosom Med 1987; 49:397–409.
5. Gelfand MM. Estrogen-androgen hormone replacement. In: Swartz DP, ed. Hormone Replacement Therapy. London: Williams & Wilkins, 1992: 221–234.
6. Ettinger B, Genant HK, Steiger P. Low-dosage micronized 17-β estradiol prevents bone loss in postmenopausal women. Am J Obstet Gynecol 1992; 166:479–488.
7. Gelfand MM, Wiita B. Androgen and estrogen-androgen hormone replacement therapy: a review of the safety literature, 1941 to 1996. Clin Ther 1997; 19:383–404.
8. Gelfand MM. Sexuality among older women. J Womens Health Gend-Based Med 2000; 9(supp.1):S15–S20.

9. Davis S. Testosterone and sexual desire in women. J Sex Edu Ther 2000; 25:25–32.
10. Davis SR, McCloud P. Testosterone enhances estradiol's effects on postmenopausal bone density and sexuality. Maturitas 1995; 21:227–236.
11. Sarrel PM, Dobay B. Estrogen and estrogen-androgen replacement in postmenopausal women dissatisfied with estrogen-only therapy: sexual behaviour and neuroendocrine responses. J Reprod Med 1998;43: 847–856.
12. Shifren J, Braunstein G. Transdermal testosterone treatment in women with impaired sexual function after oophorectomy. N Engl J Med 2000; 343:682–688.
13. Burger HG, Hailes J. The management of persistent menopausal symptoms with estradiol-testosterone implants clinical, lipid and hormonal results. Maturitas 1984; 6:351–358.
14. Watts NB, Notelovitz M. Comparison of oral estrogens and estrogen plus androgen on bone mineral density, menopausal symptoms, and lipid-lipoprotein profiles in surgical menopause (published erratum appears in Obstet Gynecol 1995; 85(5 pt 1):668], Obstet Gynecol 1995; 85:529–537.
15. Simon JA, Klaiber E. Double-blind comparison of two doses of estrogen and estrogen-androgen therapy in naturally postmenopausal women: neuroendocrine, psychological and psychosomatic effects. Fertil Steril 1996; 66:S71.
16. Longcope C, Baker RS. Androgen and estrogen dynamics in women with vertebral crush. Maturitas 1984; 6:309–318.
17. Johansson C, Mellstrom D. Reproductive factors as predictors of bone density and fractures in women at the age of 70. Maturitas 1993; 17: 39–50.
18. Morishima A, Grumbach MM. Aromatase deficiency in male and female siblings caused by a novel mutation in the physiological role of estrogens. J Clin Endocrinol Metab 1995; 80:3689–3698.
19. Raisz LG, Wiita B. Comparison of the effects of estrogen alone and estrogen plus androgen on the biochemical markers of bone formation and resorption in postmenopausal women. J Clin Endocrinol Metab 1996; 81:37–43.
20. Savvas M, Studd JW. Increase in bone mass after one year of percutaneous estradiol and testosterone implants in postmenopausal women who have previously received long-term oral estrogens. Br J Obstet Gynaecol 1992; 99:757–760.
21. Barrett-Connor E, Timmons C. Interim safety analysis of a two-year

study comparing oral estrogen-androgen and conjugated estrogens in surgically menopaused women. The estratest working group. J Womens Health 1996; 5:593–602.

22. Gelfand MM. The role of androgen replacement therapy for postmenopausal women. Contemp OB/GYN 2000, Feb:1–5.

23. Honoré EK, Williams JK. Methyltestosterone does not diminish the beneficial effects of estrogen replacement therapy on coronary artery reactivity in cynomolgus monkeys. Menopause 1996; 3:20–26.

24. Worboys S, Kotsopoulos D. Evidence that testosterone therapy may improve endothelium-dependent and -independent vasodilation in postmenopausal women already receiving estrogen. J Clin Endocrinol Metab 2001; 86:158–161.

25. Adamson D, Webb C, Collins P. Esterified estrogens combined with methyltestosterone improve emotional well-being in postmenopausal women with chest pain and normal coronary angiograms. Menopause 2001; 8:233–238.

26. Gelfand MM, Ferenczy A. Endometrial response to estrogen-androgen stimulation. In: Hammond CB, Haseltine FP, eds. Menopause: Evaluation, Treatment and Health Concerns. New York: Alan R. Liss, 1989: 29–40.

27. Lovell CW. Breast cancer incidence with parenteral estradiol and testosterone replacement therapy (abstr). Menopause 1994; 1:150.

28. Poulin R, Baker D, Labrie F. Androgens inhibit basal and estrogen-induced cell proliferation in the ZR-75-1 human breast cancer cell line. Breast Cancer Res Treat 1988; 12:213–225.

29. Kellokumpu-Lehtinen P, Huovinen R. Hormonal treatment of advanced breast cancer. A randomized trial of tamoxifen versus nandrolone decanoate. Cancer 1987; 60:2376–2381.

30. Marks LE. Sensory perception and ovarian secretions. In: Naftolein F, DeCherney AH, Guttmann JN, Sarrel PM, eds. Ovarian Secretions and Cardiovascular and Neurological Function. New York: Raven Press, 1990:223-238.

31. Hammond J, Le Q, Goodyer C, Gelfand MM, Trifiro M, Leblanc A. Testosterone-mediated neuroprotection through the androgen receptor in human primary neurons. J Neurochem 2001; 77:1–9.

4

Hormone Replacement Therapy and Cancer

Elene Strates and Charles C. Coddington
Denver Health Medical Center and University of Colorado, Denver, Colorado, U.S.A.

I. INTRODUCTION

The benefits of hormone replacement therapy (HRT) have been clearly and monumentally established, and have included improvement in postmenopausal symptoms such as hot flashes, dyspareunia, vaginal dryness, sleep disturbances, and mental acuity as well as vast health benefits in decreasing the risk of heart disease and osteoporosis [1]. Although many postmenopausal women would benefit from the reduction of cardiovascular disease and osteoporosis, and millions are interested in alleviation of their symptoms, the concern about the possible medical risks are paramount and prevent many women from initiating or continuing HRT. The primary reason that women shun estrogens during the perimenopausal and postmenopausal years has been that they believe that their risk of breast cancer is vastly elevated with the use of HRT. The overwhelming belief that breast cancer is the most pervasive health concern of all women further drives women away from HRT. Few women neither hear nor understand the controversy about whether HRT is even associated with breast cancer risk. Certainly, no one has shown that estrogens can cause breast cancer, although other adenocarcinomas such as endometrial cancer have had a large association with unopposed estrogen use. However, the effect of estrogens and progestins on cancers, even endometrial cancers, that have already been treated is complex. Early observational data have now shown that HRT is not associated with an increased risk of recurrence of breast, ovarian, or endometrial cancers.

The incidence of some adenocarcinomas such as colon cancers seem to be reduced with the use of HRT, whereas other squamous cancers, such as cervical cancer, are not affected by either endogenous estrogens or HRT.

In this chapter, we will discuss the associations between HRT use and the subsequent risk of developing cancer, as well as the possible effect of HRT on women who have had gynecological malignancies in the past.

II. THE RISK OF ENDOMETRIAL CANCER IN WOMEN TAKING HRT

For more than 25 years a clear association has been established between the use of unopposed estrogens in any form and the risk of developing endometrial carcinoma [2–5]. In contrast, addition of progestins of a certain dose and duration can not only significantly reduce, but also may even eliminate the risk of developing estrogen-induced endometrial cancer [6–8]. In the early 1970s, several investigators found a relative risk of developing endometrial carcinoma to be between 7.6 and 4.5 as compared to women who did not take unopposed estrogens [2,5]. This risk increased with duration of use and with increasing dose of estrogens. Significantly, the increased risk may persist for many years after estrogen therapy is stopped.

Grady conducted a meta-analysis of 30 previous studies (3). The relative risk for acquiring endometrial cancer was 2.3 (95% confidence interval [CI] 2.1–2.5) for women who had ever used unopposed estrogen compared to women who had never used estrogens. Even at relatively low doses of estrogens, such as conjugated equine estrogens (CEE) of 0.3 mg/day, the risk of endometrial cancer was elevated at 3.9 (95% CI, 1.6–9.5). Furthermore, as the dose and duration of estrogens increased, so did the risk. Even for less than 1 year of use, there was an increased risk of 1.4 (95% CI, 1.0–1.8). After 10 years of use, the relative risk (RR) increased to 9.5 (95% CI, 7.4–12.3). It is also suggested that the neoplastic process induced by estrogen might continue for many years after estrogen is stopped. After 5 years of discontinuing estrogen use, these women continued to have a significant increased risk of endometrial cancer with an RR of 2.3 (95% CI, 1.8–3.1). However, most of these cancers were of early stage (RR 4.2 vs. late-stage cancer at 1.4) and tended to be noninvasive (RR for noninvasive cancer was 6.2 vs. 3.8 for estrogen users with invasive cancer) as substantiated in other studies [9,10]. Perhaps endometrial cancers associated with the use of exogenous estrogens arise from a different neoplastic source than those that arise de novo [11].

Although most of these investigations in this comprehensive meta-analysis were observational studies, the risk of endometrial cancer with unopposed estrogen was seen in almost all of the studies and with increasing the dose and duration of estrogen. Thus, this association seems to be consistent with biological causality.

Once it was recognized that estrogen alone could have an overwhelming effect on acquiring endometrial cancer, progestins were added in order to stabilize the endometrium and reduce the risk of uterine cancer. Progestins can reduce the concentration of cytosolic estrogen receptors, and in a dose-dependent fashion, produce a secretory pattern of endometrial histology [12]. At least 10 days of progestin is required each month in order to have a consistent secretory pattern and to reduce the risk of hyperplasia [13]. Clinically, the number of days that progestin is given seems to be paramount [6,14,15]. In a large case-controlled study of 791 controls of women with endometrial cancer who did not take hormones vs. 833 women with cancer who took daily estrogen with cyclic progestin for less than 10 days of each month, the adjusted odds ratio (OR) was 1.87 (95% CI, 1.32–2.65) for endometrial cancer [6]. These women still had a significant risk for endometrial cancer, although it was still somewhat lower than that for women who took estrogens alone who had an OR 2.17 (95% CI, 1.91–2.47). In this study and several others, those who took daily combined HRT have been shown to have a lower risk of endometrial cancer than those on a cyclic regimen, essentially abolishing the risk of endometrial cancer

(OR 1.07; 95% CI, 0.8–1.43) [15]. It is noteworthy that in at least one large case-controlled study of 687 subjects conducted in Sweden even 10 days of progestin in a cyclic regimen did not confer absolute endometrial protection [14]. The adjusted odds ratio was 2.0 with an 95% CI of 1.4–2.7. In studies which stratified their data by the number of years that cyclic HRT was used, increasing the duration of use significantly increased the odds ratio in some studies but not others [6,14,16,17].

Although there is concern that some studies have shown an increased risk of endometrial cancer in patients who use a 10-day regimen of progestin per month, all studies to date have shown a protective effect of continuous combined HRT. Odds ratios for continuous progestins with daily estrogens are constantly nonsignificant and range from 0.7 (95% CI, 0.4–1.0) in the Swedish study of 682 patients to an OR of 1.07 (95% CI, 0.8–1.43) in the U.S. study conducted by Pike [6,14]. The overwhelming protective effect of daily estrogen with daily progestin continues even as the duration of use increases.

On a short-term basis (less than 3 years of use), most studies allow for cyclic HRT, in that this regimen does not seem to increase the risk of endometrial cancer. If patients are to continue with HRT, a continuous combined regimen of daily estrogen with daily progestin seems to confer better endometrial protection. Typically, women in the perimenopausal transition continue to have some irregular cycles. They are initially placed on a cyclic regimen of HRT in order to reduce the incidence of irregular bleeding. After a year or two most of these women will no longer have any viable follicles and thus no longer have spontaneous vaginal bleeding. At that time, placing these patients on a daily regimen is clinically and epidemeologically warranted.

With the myriad progestins and combination therapies now available, few patients with a uterus who need and choose HRT should take unopposed estrogens. Certainly the risk of endometrial cancer in this setting is substantial and well established. Yearly endometrial sampling has been advocated in this setting, but especially in the United States, where more potent estrogens are generally used, yearly endometrial biopsy may not detect all precancerous lesions before they have developed into cancer. The use of unopposed estrogens should be discouraged.

III. HORMONE REPLACEMENT THERAPY IN ENDOMETRIAL CANCER PATIENTS

During the last 15 years, hormone replacement therapy given to women with a previous history of endometrial cancer has slowly gained acceptance, especially among gynecological oncologists. Despite the fact that many retrospective studies have shown substantial benefit from HRT without any increase in recurrence [9,18–21], many clinicians have found it difficult to prescribe HRT to women with a prior history of endometrial cancer, because estrogen therapy is a primary risk factor of acquiring cancer of the uterus [3]. In addition, individual factors known to increase endogenous estrogens or the lifetime exposure to estrogens, such as obesity, age at menarche and menopause, age at first pregnancy, or anovulation have all been shown to increase the risk of endometrial cancer [22]. The relative lack of progesterone can lead not only to endometrial overgrowth and a thick endometrial lining, but also to a predominance of an estradiol environment, which promotes cell growth and division. In primate endometrium, progesterone is well known to inhibit estrogen receptors, decrease epidermal growth factor (EGF) gene expression, induce expression of transforming growth factor beta-2 (TGFβ-2), and thus reduce proliferation of the endometrium [23,24]. Theoretically, Suriano and others have proposed that estrogen may act as a promoter to cells that are susceptible to DNA damage by increasing cell division, but estrogens may not have any effect on neoplastic endometrial cells [21,25,26].

Although data are limited, the best study thus far describing the use of estrogens following treatment for endometrial cancer has been a retrospective case-controlled investigation of 150 patients [21]. Most patients initiated HRT within 6 months of cancer treatment. Approximately 86% had stage I disease in both the controls and those who took HRT. However, approximately 27% of patients in each group were deemed to have high-risk tumor profiles, such as nuclear grade III, greater than 49% myometrial involvement, and cervical extension, and required postoperative adjunctive radiotherapy after pelvic lymph node dissection. After a mean follow-up of about 7 years, women who took HRT had a substantial reduction in their recurrence rates as compared to nonusers. There were 11 recurrences in the control group

(14%) compared to 2 recurrences in the HRT group (1%), which was statistically significant ($P < 0.006$). Half of the patients took a combination of estrogen with progesterone, because there is a theoretical reduction of endometrial cell proliferation with the addition of progesterone. However, whether women took estrogens alone or an estrogen and progesterone combination did not alter the results.

At this time, retrospective studies have shown that HRT following treatment for endometrial cancer does not increase the chance of recurrence [18–20]. However, all of these studies have been small and many of them had a significant lag between the completion of therapy for endometrial cancer and the initiation of HRT. Certainly the type of estrogen prescribed has not been consistent nor recorded in some cases, and in other studies patients who took progestins were combined with those who took estrogens alone. Many of these studies lacked a control group and often included all of the histological types of endometrial cancers as a block. Currently, the Gynecologic Oncology Group is conducting a prospective randomized clinical trial of estrogen replacement therapy in patients with stage I and II endometrial adenocarcinoma. To discern sufficient power, more than 1000 thousand patients will be enrolled in each arm, with follow-up over 5 years. Until this study is completed, the current evidence supports the possible use of HRT in women who have been treated for endometrial cancer and may derive specific benefit from this treatment.

IV. THE RISK OF BREAST CANCER IN WOMEN TAKING HRT

For most women taking or considering HRT, the fear that hormones may increase the likelihood of acquiring breast cancer is of primary concern [27]. Numerous studies of compliance with HRT have repeatedly shown that the fear of breast cancer is one of the primary reasons for stopping HRT, despite the well-recognized benefits of elevation of perimenopausal symptoms, reduction in the risk of heart disease and osteoporosis, and decrease in overall mortality [1,28]. Clinically and scientifically, there has been little agreement about whether or not HRT indeed increases the risk of breast cancer in the vast majority of women who take hormones in the perimenopausal or postmenopausal era.

Although some studies have shown an increased risk of developing (or detecting) breast cancer, these patients uniformly tend to have early tumors with little evidence of metastasis [29]. Furthermore, these women tend to have a smaller chance of dying than women who are not taking HRT, despite being diagnosed with breast cancer [29,30]. Certainly in many studies, the possibility of detection bias (as reflected in the higher rate of mammography in these patients) may explain the modest increased risk of breast cancer as well as the observation that these patients have early disease [31]. Some have argued that if estrogens and progestins through complex mechanisms caused breast cancer, we would expect that women currently taking HRT should have aggressive tumors with a higher distribution of metastasis. This result has not been borne out of any of the current observational studies. Other cancers that are hormone dependent also do not show aggressive tumors with increasing duration of HRT use. Although endometrial cancer is well known to be associated with unopposed estrogen use, these cancers tend to be early and do not show metastasis. Perhaps gonadal steroids act as promoters rather than initiators of cancers in the breast and endometrium.

Some studies have shown an increase in breast cancer with duration of use, whereas others have not [32–41]. In the large combined reanalysis of 51 studies conducted by the Imperial Cancer Research Fund, the risk of breast cancer increased with duration of use, but in an inconsistent manner, such that there was an increased risk of breast cancer at 5 years and above 15 years not at 10 years (RR at 5 years 1.19; 99% CI, 1.129–1.251, RR at 10 years was 1.09 with 99% CI 1.003–1.177, with RR at greater than 15 years at 1.459–1.701) [32]. The literature abounds with such inconsistencies, perhaps reflecting the highly complex effect of estrogens and progestins on the breast.

Breast tumors are known to have large intracellular concentrations of estrogens that may not be reflected in the serum. The modulation and biological effect of these local estrogens is probably more complex than has been imagined. As an example, during the last 10 years two estrogen receptors have been identified, whereas, previously only one was known. Exogenous estrogens and progestins down regulate their receptors and cause proliferation of the breast in the nonhuman primate [42]. The potential for individual tissue differences in estrogen and progestin metabolism, binding, and damage to cellular DNA is immense. Body weight, diet, and exercise may also further modulate endogenous estrogen function. These "lifestyle" factors may include the increased production of estrone in adipose tissue or the effect of phytoestrogens on estrogen receptors. In addition, the effects from aromatase inhibitors and enzyme-modulating therapy must be studied further.

In more than 50 observational studies that have been conducted over the last 50 years, there has not been any consistent evidence that HRT increases the risk of breast cancer [32–41]. In some studies, a family history of breast cancer increased the risk of acquiring breast cancer [37,39], but in others it did not [32,33,40]. In one study, which identified the specific hormone regimen that was used, the addition of a cyclic progestin to estrogen seemed to increase the risk of breast cancer (RR 1.38; 95% CI, 1.13–1.68), although daily combined estrogen and progestin did not (RR 1.09; 95% CI, 0.88–1.35) [43]. However other studies showed an increase in RR with daily combined HRT [35]. At this point, because the data are inconsistent, most researchers agree that if there is an increased risk of breast cancer, this effect is small and probably only limited to a small high-risk population which has not yet been identified.

V. THE RISK OF BREAST CANCER IN WOMEN TAKING SELECTIVE ESTROGEN RECEPTOR MODULATORS

Estrogen receptor agonists/antagonists occupy the estrogen receptor in a variety of tissues. Raloxifine is the only SERM, except tamoxifen, that is currently available in the United States. In 2001, a follow-up report was published on the multiple outcomes of raloxifene evaluation (MORE) trial [44]. In this study, 7705 women were enrolled whose mean age was 66.5 years (19 years postmenopausal) to investigate the osteoporotic effect of raloxifene and the incidence of breast cancer. There were 61 invasive breast cancers. This was a 72% reduction and a relative risk of 0.28 (95% CI, 0.17–0.46). This effect was strictly seen in estrogen receptor positive breast cancers. With increasing use of up to 4 years, there continued to be a reduction in risk. As previously reported, raloxifene did not cause vaginal bleeding or endometrial cancer compared to placebo. Raloxifene has been shown to increase bone density, but has no effect on climacteric symptoms or on vaginal atrophy [45]. It may also reduce the chance of cardiovascular disease through its favorable effect on serum lipids.

Thus, in some patients who do not want to take any risk of promoting breast cancer, raloxifene will be their first hormonal choice in reducing the risk or treating osteoporosis. Whether the reduction in breast cancer is seen in those patients with BRAC mutation is not known. Certainly raloxifene, because it does not address women's symptoms, will not be useful in a vast number of patients.

VI. HORMONE REPLACEMENT THERAPY IN WOMEN WITH A HISTORY OF BREAST CANCER

As noted earlier, the relationship between breast cancer and estrogen or progestins is complex and contradictory. Estrogens and progestins in tissue culture can promote and inhibit growth of the normal breast. In established cultures of breast cancer, the actions of estrogen are even more confusing. At low doses, estrogen can stimulate growth, whereas in higher doses estrogens may inhibit growth [46]. Adding more complexity to the effect of steroids in this system is the observation that estrogen and progesterone receptors may be expressed in various amounts before and after breast cancer therapy, thus they may further modulate the effect of exogenous or endogenous estrogens on the breast or even on micrometastases. Although a growing body of evidence has not shown a clear deleterious effect of HRT on initiating new breast cancer, many clinicians are reluctant to prescribe HRT to women who have already been treated for this malignancy, because estrogen receptor modulators such as tamoxifen have been clearly shown to reduce the risk of subsequent recurrence or progression of the disease [47].

Over the last 5 years, several observational studies have not shown an increased recurrence of breast cancer in those women who took HRT for relief of menopausal symptoms after treatment for their cancers. The meta-analysis completed by Col is indicative of the conclusions of most of these studies [48]. Eleven studies were included over the 33-year period between 1966 and 1999. Seventeen studies were excluded either for redundant data, failure to report recurrences, failure to report a sample size, or reporting only on ductal carcinoma in situ (DCIS) and not on invasive breast cancer. The relative risk of having a recurrent breast cancer in 669 women who took HRT as compared to 1078 women who did not was 0.82 (95% CI, = 0.58–1.15). This suggests that HRT use by women with a history of invasive breast cancer does not significantly increase the risk of recurrence. Most women in these studies had been treated for early stage I or II breast cancer at least 2 years before initiating HRT, and then had taken HRT for an average of 22 months, primarily as symptomatic relief from the menopause. As with all studies in the literature, it is difficult to generalize these data to all breast cancer patients, because women were not randomized and the type of breast cancer or HRT that was taken was not reported.

Most women who take HRT after treatment for their breast cancer do so for relief of their immediate perimenopausal symptoms such as vaginal dryness or hot flushes. Thus, relatively few studies have reported on type of HRT that was used, such as estrogen alone or combined HRT, much less the exact dose or class of hormone. In 2001, O'Meara reported on 869 breast cancer survivors, 174 who took HRT as compared to 695 who did not [47]. In this case-controlled retrospective study, 79% of women took estrogens alone without a progestin. The adjusted relative risk of breast cancer in women who took HRT was 0.50 (95% CI, = 0.30–0.85), thus showing a decreased incidence of recurrence in women who took HRT as compared to those who did not. This relative reduction in risk was the same whether patients took estrogen alone or estrogen with progestin.

On a short-term basis, HRT seems to be safe in the breast cancer survivor with early stage I and II breast cancer. Given that combination HRT may increase the risk of acquiring breast cancer in healthy women, and that HRT is known to increase the density of the breast and possibly reduce the ability to detect early secondary primary tumors or recurrences, women who have been treated for breast cancer who elect to use HRT should do so with some caution. It is reasonable to coordinate therapy with all care providers.

VII. THE RISK OF CERVICAL CANCER IN WOMEN TAKING HRT

The vast majority of squamous cervical cancers are associated with infection and, specifically, human papillomaviruses (HPVs) [49]. Estrogen and progestin can enhance the ability of HPV to transform benign epithelial cells into cancer by upregulating the estrogen receptor and increasing the rate of transformation [49,50]. Most epidemiological studies however have not shown an increased risk of cervical cancer in women taking estrogens alone or estrogens with progestins [51,52]. In 1997, Parazzini published a case-controlled study of 645 women with cervical cancer and 749 controls [51]. Forty women with cervical cancer had taken estrogens (of these, 35 had taken estrogens alone), whereas 85 controls had taken hormones (80 had taken estrogens alone). When adjusted for known social and demographic factors such as age, social class, parity, number of sexual partners, oral contraceptive use, smoking, menopausal status, and screening with lifetime number of cervical smears, the adjusted odds ratio was 0.5 (95% CI, 0.3–0.8). This relationship did not change with increasing the number of years of estrogen replacement therapy (OR 0.5; 95% CI, 0.2–1.0, for use greater than 12 months). This study is limited not only by the small number of women who took estrogens (and even fewer who took combined HRT), but also because the type of cervical cancer was not specified. The authors included both squamous and adenocarcinomas. Twenty-five percent of the cancers were not histologically specified at all. It is possible that adenocarcinomas and squamous cancers of the cervix are promoted by different factors. Adenocarcinomas may proliferate with HRT use, whereas squamous cancers may not. In a study of 124 patients with adenocarcinoma of the cervix, 13 had used hormones, whereas 109 had not [52]. With these small numbers, the odds ratio was 2.1, showing a possible increased risk of adenocarcinoma of the cervix with use of estrogens, although the confidence interval did cross 1 (95% CI, 0.95–4.6). However, this was again a small study group and as the duration of use increased, the odds ratios actually decreased. As the incidence of adenocarcinomas of the cervix continues to rise, we will need to be diligent about identifying any associations that may exist.

Although there is a paucity of data of women taking combined HRT of both estrogen and progestin, it seems that hormones do not play a significant risk in promoting cervical cancer. Information from studies of oral contraceptive use does not support an increase risk of cervical cancer when these cohorts are adjusted for age, number of sexual partners, age at first intercourse, and cervical sampling [53]. At this time, hormone replacement therapy does not seem to be associated with an increased risk of cervical cancer. Caution must be taken, however, because only a handful of studies have been published, all of which have had relatively few patients.

VIII. HORMONE REPLACEMENT THERAPY IN WOMEN WITH A HISTORY OF CERVICAL CANCER

Although gonadal steroids are known to affect the cervix, there is no clinical evidence that hormones are associated with the development or recurrence of squamous cervical cancer. Until the appearance of Ploch's study in 1985, routine ovarian preservation was not the norm even in stage I and II cervical cancer patients [54]. Hormone replacement therapy was felt to be a "hazard" and was also withheld. Eighty patients in Ploch's study were treated with cyclic progestins and daily estrogens and 40 patients did not receive HRT. At 5 years, 80% of the HRT group had survived, while 65% of the patients were alive who did not take HRT. This difference was not statistically significant. Similarly, the number of recurrences and the time from cancer treatment to recurrence were not significantly different. Preservation of ovarian function and routine use of HRT has now become the accepted practice in women who have been treated for squamous cervical cancers.

IX. THE RISK OF OVARIAN CANCER IN WOMEN TAKING HRT

The effect of estradiol and gonadotropins, such as follicle stimulating hormone (FSH), on the ovary are complex. Both hormones have been shown to promote growth of ovarian carcinomas in vitro in varying concentrations (55). Gonadotropins in low serum concentrations have been shown to be associated with a higher risk of ovarian cancer in postmenopausal patients [56], whereas use of oral contraceptives in women of reproductive age has been shown to reduce gonadotropins and the risk of ovarian cancer by more than 50% (53). Exogenous estrogens may promote ovarian cancer by occupying estrogen receptors in the cytosol and nucleus, and thus increasing malignant transformation over time. Short-term studies on HRT have not shown a consistent effect on the rate of ovarian cancer mortality or incidence [54–56]. However, recent long-term studies show an increase in deaths from ovarian cancer in those women using HRT for more than 10 years [57,58].

Rodriguez reported on the American Cancer Society's Cancer Prevention Study II, which was a prospective study of postmenopausal women [57]. Out of 944 women who died from ovarian cancer, 255 who had ever used estrogens had a relative risk of dying from ovarian cancer of 1.23 (95% CI, 1.06–1.43) when adjusted for race, duration of oral contraceptive use, number of live births, age at menopause, body mass index, age at menarche, and tubal ligation. In this study, as in most studies to date, the type of HRT was not specified with regard to type of estrogen or use of progestin. Because this cohort was initially recruited in 1982, many of these women were taking unopposed estrogens. For women who took HRT for less than 10 years, the RR was not significant, but for women who took HRT for more than 10 years, the RR was 2.20 (95% CI, 1.53–3.17). Thus, in the short term, HRT did not increase the risk of dying from ovarian cancer, but with many years of estrogen use there seems to be a significant increased risk of mortality from ovarian cancer. Similar data were found in a collaborative reanalysis of four case-controlled studies in Europe [58] with an RR of 1.71 (95% CI, 1.30–2.25), and in a meta-analysis in the United States [56] (RR 1.4 95% CI, 0.74–2.5) Because most women are currently taking HRT in the combined form of both estrogen and a progestin, it is difficult to counsel women regarding their risk of ovarian cancer at this time. Certainly in the short term, when women use estrogens for less than 10 years, there does not seem to be a significant risk of ovarian cancer.

X. HORMONE REPLACEMENT THERAPY IN WOMEN WITH A HISTORY OF OVARIAN CANCER

The number of studies of HRT in women who have been treated for ovarian cancer are few, but encouraging. Theoretically, ovarian carcinomas have been thought to be hormonally dependent, but even though estrogen and progesterone receptors have been found in these neoplasms, the association with survival has not been consistent [59,60]. A randomized prospective study of estrogen replacement therapy was reported in 1999 [61]. Out of a total of 130 patients, 59 were randomized to estrogen alone and 66 to no treatment. After following these women for at least 4 years, there was no significant difference in either the disease-free interval or overall survival between women who took HRT or those who did not take estrogens (34 months vs. 27 months, respectively, for disease-free interval, and 44 months vs. 34 months for overall survival).

Other retrospective studies showed similar results (62). At least in the short term, estrogens may be beneficial to women with ovarian cancer. Caution must be taken however, because in healthy women who use HRT on a long-term basis (for more than 10 years), a significant increase in risk has been found.

XI. THE RISK OF COLORECTAL CANCER IN WOMEN TAKING HRT

Although excess bile acids are thought to be direct carcinogens to the colon [63], estrogens have long been recognized to decrease the synthesis and secretion of bile acids, thus conferring a protective effect and reducing the risk of colon cancer. Since this hypothesis was first postulated in 1980 by McMichael and Potter [64], more than 12 studies have confirmed that using HRT decreases the risk of colorectal cancer [65–87]. The protective effect of HRT has been strengthened by a continued reduction in the development of colorectal cancer with an increase in the number of years that HRT was used. Although a handful of studies have shown no reduction in colorectal cancer with the use of HRT, none have shown an increased risk.

In 1998, Fernandez combined the data from two large Italian case-controlled studies [87]. There was a 42% reduction in colorectal cancer for women who had ever used HRT, even when adjusted for a variety of confounders including age, diet, smoking, alcohol consumption, family history, and body mass index (OR = 0.58; 95% CI, 0.44–0.76). As women continued to use HRT the risk of colorectal cancer continued to decrease, and thus there was a clear decline in risk with duration of use (OR = 0.46; 95% CI, 0.26–0.81). Women with a family history of colorectal cancer had the greatest benefit (OR = 0.17) as compared to women who did not have any family members with colorectal cancer (OR = 0.58). This study was limited by the small number of women who took HRT 54 and in that the dose and type of HRT were not specified. As noted in a variety of organ systems, such as the breast or endometrium, it is possible that estrogen alone or estrogen with progesterone will result in different effects. For instance, women who take combined oral contraceptives have a 36% decrease in the incidence and mortality of colorectal cancer [88]. HRT that contains both a progestin and estrogen may indeed be most protective in reducing the risk of developing colorectal cancer. Although no studies have specifically examined the use of daily combined HRT on colorectal cancer none of the articles have shown that estrogen is associated with an increased risk of acquiring colorectal cancer.

XII. THE RISK OF THYROID CANCER IN WOMEN TAKING HRT

No prevalent hypothesis exists as to the association of thyroid cancer with reproductive hormones. However, the prevalence of thyroid cancer is increased in women of reproductive age, and therefore it is possible that estrogens and progestins may be associated with the occurrence of thyroid cancer.

In 1999, La Vecchia reported a pooled analysis of eight studies [89]; 1305 cases were studied with 2300 controls. In a comparison of 110 women who had used HRT and had thyroid cancer vs. 205 who had used HRT but did not have thyroid cancer, the odds ratio was not significant at 0.8 (95% CI, 0.6–1.1). Even with increased duration of use, the OR remained insignificant at 0.9 (95% CI, 0.6–1.3). The specific risk for combined estrogen and progestin therapy is not stratified in this study, and therefore specific risk for types of HRT can not be drawn; however, most patients took unopposed estrogens. This study indicates that HRT is not associated with thyroid cancer.

XIII. SUMMARY

Hormone replacement therapy can improve the quality of life for many women by decreasing vasomotor symptoms, providing better sleep, decreasing the incidence of fractures, alleviating vaginal dryness, and improving LDL/HDL ratio. In those women who take HRT for these reasons they have an added benefit of decreasing their risk of colorectal cancer. In the short term, ten years or less, taking combined HRT does not seem to increase the risk of acquiring the most common gynecological malignancies such as ovarian, cervical, or uterine cancers. Although many women believe that taking HRT will increase their risk of acquiring breast cancer this has not been clearly shown. Some studies show an increase in breast cancer with increasing the dose and duration of hormones while others do not. Additional information is greatly anticipated when the large multicenter Women's Health Initiative trial is concluded in 2007. For those women who have had a prior gynecologic malignancy, short term HRT provides benefits if taken for 5 years or less. Even women with previous early breast, ovarian, and endometrial cancers seem to do well and did not have an increased risk of recurrence compared to those who took nothing. Additional prospective studies are needed in this cohort of women who have already had a female malignancy and now desire HRT.

ADDENDUM

Subsequent to writing this chapter the large, well-designed Women's Health Initiative trial published a landmark report concluding that combined continuous HRT of CEE 0.625 mg and medroxyprogesterone acetate 2.5 mg increased the risk of breast cancer without reducing the risk of cardiovascular disease and surprisingly, increasing the chance of myocardial infarction and stroke [90]. Although the absolute risk was small for all these factors, between 7 to 8 additional women with each of these diseases in 10,000 patients, the study was well designed and executed. The trial was designed to evaluate an increase in acquiring disease, not merely an increase in mortality, which is a relatively late finding. Indeed after an average of 5.2 years of HRT there were no differences in mortality in those patients taking HRT versus those on placebo. However, the increased chance of acquiring breast cancer was seen after 4 years of use while that for cardiac disease was noted within the first year of HRT. This study also noted a significant reduction in the risk of acquiring colorectal cancer and hip fractures with 6 fewer cases of colorectal cancer and 5 fewer hip fractures per 10,000 women. Additionally, as expected the risk of venous thromboembolic disease was increased in the first year to 18 cases in 10,000 patient years of use. This was not surprising since all types of estrogens, including HRT and oral contraceptives, have long been known to increase the risk of deep vein thrombosis and pulmonary embolus. The significance of this study is that it was a large double blind randomized trial of over 16,000 healthy postmenopausal women between the ages of 50 and 74. At least in this age group, when the incidence of breast cancer inclines sharply, it seems prudent to offer combined daily HRT to primarily alleviate vasomotor and genitourinary symptoms for a shorter time. There may be patients, of course, who have additional risks factors, such as a strong family history of colorectal cancer, in whom a further individualized prolonged regimen of HRT may be considered.

REFERENCES

1. Lobo RA. Benefit and risk of estrogen replacement therapy. Am J Obstet Gynecol 1995; 173:982–989.
2. Smith DC, Prentice R, Thompson DJ. Association of exogenous estrogen and endometrial carcinoma. N Engl J Med 1975; 293:1164–1167.
3. Grady D, Gebretsadik T, Kerlikowske K, Ernster V, Petitti D. Hormone replacement therapy and endometrial cancer risk: a meta-analysis. Obstet Gynecol 1995; 85:304–313.
4. Hulka BS, Kaufman DG, Fowler, WC, Grimson, RC, Greenberg, BG.

Predominance of early endometrial cancers after long-term estrogen use. JAMA 1980; 244:2419–2422.

5. Ziel HK, Finkle WD. Increased risk of endometrial carcinoma among users of conjugated estrogens. N Engl J Med 1975; 293:1167–1170.

6. Pike MC, Peters RK, Cozen W, Probst-Hensch NM, Felix JC, Wan PC, Mack TM. Estrogen-progestin replacement therapy and edometrial cancer. J Natl Cancer Inst 1997; 89:1110–1116.

7. Whitehead M, Lobo RA. Consensus conference: Progestagen use in postmenopausal women. Lancet 1988; 2:1243–1244.

8. Persson I, Adami H, Bergkvist L, Lindgren A, Pettersson B, Hoover R, Schairer C. Risk of endometrial cancer after treatment with oestrogens alone or in conjunction with progestogens: results of a prospective study. Br Med J 1989; 298:147–151.

9. Elwood JM, Boyes DA. Clinical and pathological features and survival of endometrial cancer patients in relation to prior use of estrogens. Gyn Onc 1980; 10:173–187.

10. Collins J, Donner A, Allen LH, Adams O. Oestrogen use and survival in endometrial cancer. Lancet 1980; 2:961–964.

11. Ryan KJ, Berkowitz RS, Borbien RL, Duraif A. Kistner's Gynecology and Women's Health. 7th ed. St. Louis: Mosby, 1999:133.

12. Gibbons WE, Moyer DL, Lobo RA. Biochemical and histologic effects of sequential estrogen/progestin therapy on the endometrium of postmenopausal women. Am J Obstet Gynecol 1986; 154:456–461.

13. Woodruff JD, Pickar JH. Incidence of endometrial hyperplasia in postmenopausal women taking conjugated estrogens (Premarin) with medroxyprogesterone acetate or conjugated estrogens alone. The Menopause Study Group. Am J Obstet Gynecol 1994; 170:1213–1223.

14. Weiderpass E, Adami HO, Baron JA, Magnusson C, Bergstrom R, Lindgren A, Correia N, Persson I. Risk of endometrial cancer following estrogen replacement with and without progestins. J Natl Cancer Inst 1999; 92: 1131–1132.

15. Jain MG, Rohan TE, Howe GR. Hormone replacement therapy and endometrial cancer in Ontario, Canada. J Clin Epidemiol 2000; 53:385–391.

16. Beresford SA. Risk of endometrial cancer in relation to use of oestrogen combined with cyclic progestagen therapy in postmenopausal women. Lancet 1997; 349:458–461.

17. Persson I. Estrogens in the causation of breast, endometrial, and ovarian cancers–evidence hypothesis from epidemiological findings. J Steroid Biochem Mol Biol 2000; 74:357–364.

18. Creasman W, Henderson D, Hinshaw W, Clarke-Pearson D. Estrogen replacement in the patient treated for endometrial cancer. Obstet Gynecol 1986; 67:326–330.
19. Lee R, Burke T, Park R. Estrogen replacement therapy following treatment for stage I endometrial carcinoma. Gynecol Oncol 1990; 36:189–191.
20. Chapman J DiSaia P, Osann K, Roth P, Gilotte D, Berman M. Estrogen replacement in surgical stage I and II endometrial cancer survivors. Am J Obstet Gynecol 1996; 175:1195–2000.
21. Suriano KA, McHale M, McLaren CE, Li K, Re A, DiSia PJ. Estrogen replacement therapy in endometrial cancer patients: a matched control study. Obstet Gynecol 2001; 97:555–560.
22. Parazzino F, La Vecchia C, Bocciolone L, Franceschi S. The epidemiology of endometrial cancer. Gynecol Oncol 1991; 41:1–16.
23. Ace CI, Okulicz WC. Differential gene regulation by estrogen and progesterone in the primate endometrium. Mol Cell Endocrinol 1995; 115:95–103.
24. Clarke CL, Sutherland, RL. Progestin regulation of cellular proliferation. Endocr Rev 1990; 11:266–301.
25. Samsioe G. The endometrium: effects of estrogen and estrogen-progesterone replacement therapy. Int J Fertil Menopausal Study 1994; 39:84–92.
26. Li SF, Shiozawa T, Nakayama K, Nikaido T, Fujii S. Stepwise abnormality of sex steroids, hormone receptors, tumor suppressor gene products (p53 and Rb), and cyclin E in uterine endometroid carcinoma. Cancer 1996; 77:321–329.
27. Col NF, Eckman MH, Koras RH. Patient specific decisions about hormone replacement therapy in postmenopausal women. JAMA 1997; 277:1140–1143.
28. Schairere C, Adami HO, Hoover R, Persson I. Cause-specific mortality in women receiving hormone replacement therapy. Epidemiology 1997; 8:59–65
29. Bonnier P, Bessenay F, Sasco AJ, Beedassy B, Lejeune C, Romain S, Charpin C, Piana L, Martin PM. Impact of menopausal hormone-replacement therapy on clinical and laboratory characteristics of breast cancer. Int J Cancer 1998; 79:278–282
30. Grodstein F, Stampfer MJ, Colditz GA, Willett WC, Manson JE, Joffee M, Rosner B, Fuchs C, Hankinson SE, Hunter DJ, Hennekens CH, Speizer FE. Postmenopausal hormone replacement therapy and mortality. N Engl J Med 1997; 336:1769–1775.

31. Grodstein F, Stampfer MJ, Manson JE, Colditz GA, Willett WC, Rosner B, Speizer FE, Hennekens CH. Postmenopausal estrogen and progestin use and the risk of cardiovascular disease. N Engl J Med 1996; 335: 453–461.

32. Collaborative Group on Hormonal Factors in Breast Cancer. Breast cancer and hormone replacement therapy: collaborative reanalysis of data from 51 epidemiological studies of 52,705 women with breast cancer and 108,411 women without breast cancer. Lancet 1997; 350:1047–1059.

33. Lando JF, Heck KE, Brett KM. Hormone replacement therapy and breast cancer risk in a nationally representative cohort. Am J Prev Med 1999; 17:176–180.

34. Persson I, Weiderpass E, Bergkvist L, Bergstrom R, Schairer C. Risks of breast and endometrial cancer after estrogen and estrogen-progestin replacement. Cancer Causes Control 1999; 10: 253–260.

35. Magnusson C, Baron JA, Correia N, Bergstrom R, Adami HO, Persson I. Breast-cancer risk following long-term oestrogen and oestrogen-progestin-replacement therapy. Int J Cancer 1999; 81:339–344.

36. Schairer C, Lubin, J, Troisi, R, Sturgeon S, Brinton, L, Hoover, R. Menopausal estrogen and estrogen-progestin replacement therapy and breast cancer risk. JAMA 2000; 283:485–491.

37. Gapstur SM, Morrow M, Sellers TA. Hormone replacement therapy and risk of breast cancer with favorable histology. Results of the Iowa Women's Health Study. JAMA 1999; 281:2091–2097.

38. Colditz GA, Hankinson SE, Hunter DJ, Willet WC, Manson JE, Stampfer MJ, Hennekens C, Rosner B, Speizer E. The use of estrogens and progestins and the risk of breast cancer in postmenopausal women. N Engl J of Med 1995; 332:1589–1593.

39. Newcomb PA, Longnecker MP, Storer BE, Mittendorf R, Baron J, Clapp Rw, Bogdan G, Willett WC. Long-term hormone replacement therapy and risk of breast cancer in postmenopausal women. Am J Epidemiol 1995; 142:788–795.

40. Stanford JL, Weiss NS, Voigt LF, Daling JR, Habel LA, Rossing MA. Combined estrogen and progestin hormone replacement therapy in relation to risk of breast cancer in middle-age women. JAMA 1995; 274: 137–142.

41. Nachtigall MJ, Smilen SW, Nachtigall RD, Nacthigall RH, Nachtigall LE. Incidence of breast cancer in a 22-year study of women receiving estrogen-progestin replacement therapy. Ob Gyn 1992; 80:827–830.

42. Soderquist G. Effects of sex steroids on proliferation in normal mammary tissue. Ann Med 1998; 30:511–524.

43. Ross RK, Paganini-Hill A, Wan, PC, Pike PC. Effect of hormone replacement therapy on breast cancer risk: estrogen vs. estrogen plus progestin. J Natl Cancer Inst 2000; 92:328–332.

44. Cauley JA, Norton L, Lipman ME, Eckert S, Krueger KA, Purdie DW, Farrerons J, Karasik A, Mellstrom D, Wah NGK, Ng KW, Stepan JJ, Powles TJ, Morrow M, Costa A, Silfen SL, Walls EL, Schmitt H, Muchmore DB, Jordan VC, Ste-Marie LG. Continued breast cancer risk reduction in postmenopausal women treated with raloxifene: 4 year results from the MORE trial. Breast Cancer Res Treat 2001; 65:125–134.

45. Davies G, Huster WJ, Lu Y, Plouffe L, Lakshmanan M. Adverse events reported by postmenopausal women in controlled trials with raloxifene. Obstet Gynecol 1999; 93:558–565.

46. Lippman M, Bolan G, Huff K. The effects of estrogens and antiestrogens on hormone-responsive human breast cancer in long-term tissue culture. Cancer Res 1976; 36:4595–4601.

47. O'Meara ES, Rossing MA, Daling JR, Elmore JG, Barlow WE, Weiss NS. Hormone replacement therapy after a diagnosis of breast cancer in relation to recurrence and mortality. J Natl Cancer Inst 2001; 93:754–762.

48. Col NF, Hirota LK, Orr RK, Erban JK, Wong JB, Lau J. Hormone replacement therapy after breast cancer; a systematic review and quantitative assessment of risk. J Clin Oncol 2001;19: 2357–2363.

49. Pater A, Bayatpour M, Pater MM. Oncogenic transformation by human papillomavirus type 16 deoxyribonucleic acid in the presence of progesterone or progestins from oral contraceptives. Am J Obstet Gynecol 1990; 162:1099–1103.

50. Monsonego J, Magdelena H. Catalan F, Coscas Y, Zerat L, Sasike X. Estrogen and progesterone receptors in cervical human papillomavirus related lesions. Int J Cancer 1991; 485:533–539.

51. Lace JV Jr, Brinton LA, Barnes WA, Gravitt MS, Greenberg MD, Hadjimichael OC, McGowan L, Mortel R, Schwartz PE, Kurman RJ, Hildesheim A. Use of hormone replacement therapy and adenocarcinomas and squamous cell carcinomas of the uterine cervix. Gynecol Oncol 2000; 77:149–154.

52. Parazzini F. Case control study of estrogen replacement therapy and risk of cervical cancer. Br Med J 1997; 315:85–88.

53. Mishell DR Jr. Noncontraceptive benefits of oral contraceptives. J Reprod Med 1993; 38:1021–1029.

54. Ploch E. Hormonal replacement therapy in patients after cervical cancer treatment. Gynecol Oncol 1987; 26:169–177.

55. Simon WE, Albrecht M, Hansel M, Dietel M, Holzer F. Cell lines de-

rived from human ovarian carcinomas: growth stimulation by gonado-tropic and steroid hormones. J Nat Cancer Inst 1983; 70:839–848.

56. Whittemore AS, Harris R, Itnyre J. The collaborative ovarian cancer group. Characteristics relating to ovarian cancer risk: collaborative analysis of 12 US case-control studies. Am J Epidemiol 1992; 136:1184–1203.

57. Rodriguez C, Patel AV, Calle EE, Jacob EJ, Thum MJ. Estrogen replacement therapy and ovarian cancer mortality in a large prospectus of women. JAMA 2001; 285:1460–1465.

58. Negri E, Tzonou A, Beral V, Lagiou P, Trichopoulos D, Parazzino F, Franceschi S, Booth M, La Vecchia C. Hormonal therapy for menopause and ovarian cancer in a collaborative re-analysis of european studies. Int J Cancer 1999; 80:848–851.

59. Rose PJ, Reale FR, Longcope C, Hunter RE. Prognostic significance of estrogen and progesterone in ovarian epithelial cancer. Obstet Gynecol 1990; 76:258–263.

60. Severlada P, Renison U, Schemper M, Spone J, Vavra V, Salzer H. Estrogen and progesterone receptor content as a prognostic factor in advanced epithelial ovarian cancer. Br J Obstet Gynecol 1990; 97:706–712.

61. Eeles RA, Tan S, Wiltshaw E, Fryatt I, A'Hern RPA, Shepard JH, Harmer CL, Blake PR, Chilyers CED. Hormone replacement therapy and survival after surgery for ovarian cancer. Br Med J 1991; 302:259–262.

62. Guidozzi, F, Daponte A. Estrogen replacement therapy for ovarian carcinoma survivors. Cancer 1999; 86:1013 -1018.

63. Reddy BS, Watanabe K, Weisburger JH, Wynder EL. Promoting effect of bile acids on colon carcinogenesis in germ-free and conventional F344 rats. Cancer Res 1977; 37:3238–3242.

64. McMichael AJ, Potter JD. Reproduction, endogenous and exogenous sex hormones, and colon cancer: a review and hypothesis. J Natl Cancer Inst 1980; 65:1201–1207.

65. Troisi R, Schairer C, Chow W-H, Schatzkin A, Brinton LA, Fraumeni JF. A prospective study of postmenopausal hormones and risk of colo-rectal cancer. Cancer Causes Control 1997; 8:130–138.

66. Kampman E, Potter JD, Slatter ML, Caan BJ, Edwards S. Hormone replacement therapy, reproductive history, and colon cancer: a multicenter, case-control study in the United States. Cancer Causes Control 1997; 8: 146–158.

67. Grodstein F, Martinez MD, Giovannucci EL, Colditz GA, Hunter DJ,

Willett WC, Speizer FE, Stampfer MJ. Postmenopausal hormone use and colorectal cancer in the Nurses' Health Study. Am J Epidemiol 1996; 11:S63.

68. Persson I, Yuen J, Bergkvist L, Schairer C. Cancer incidence and mortality in women receiving estrogen and estrogen-progestin replacement therapy: long-term follow-up of a Swedish cohort. Int J Cancer 1996; 67:327–332.

69. Fernandez E, La Vecchia C, D'Avanzo B, Franceschi S, Negri E, Parazzini F. Oral contraceptives, hormone replacement therapy and the risk of colorectal cancer. Br J Cancer 1996; 73:1431–1435.

70. Newcomb PA, Storer BE. Postmenopausal hormone use and risk of large-bowel cancer. J Natl Cancer Inst 1995; 87:1067–1071.

71. Calle EE, Miracle-McMahill HL, Thun MJ, Heath CW. Estrogen Replacement therapy and risk of fatal colon cancer in a prospective cohort of postmenopausal women. J Natl Cancer Inst 1995; 87:517–523.

72. Jacobs EJ, White E, Weiss NS. Exogenous hormones, reproductive history, and colon cancer. Cancer Causes Control 1994; 5:359–366.

73. Gerhardsson de Verdier M, London S. Reproductive factors, exogenous female hormones, and colorectal cancer by subsite. Cancer Causes Control 1992; 3:355–360.

74. Chute CG, Willett WC, Colditz GA, Stampfer MJ, Rosner B, Speizer FE. A prospective study of reproductive history and exogenous estrogens on the risk of colorectal cancer in women. Epidemiology 1991; 2:201–207.

75. Furner SE, Davis FG, Nelson RL, Haenszel W. A case-control study of large bowel cancer and hormone exposure in women. Cancer Res 1989; 49:4936–4940.

76. Rosenberg L, Werler MM, Kaufman DW, Shapiro S. Cancer of the colon and rectum in relation to reproductive factors. Am J Epidemiol 1987; 126:760–761.

77. Folson AR, Mink PJ, Sellers TA, Hong C-P, Zheng W, Potter JD. Hormonal replacement therapy and morbidity and mortality in a prospective study of postmenopausal women. Am J Public Health 1995; 85:1128–1132.

78. Risch JA, Howe GR. Menopausal hormone use and colorectal cancer in Saskatchewan: a record linkage cohort study. Cancer Epidemiol 1995; 4:21–28.

79. Bostick RM, Potter JD, Kushi LH, Sellers TA, Steinmetz KA, McKenzie DR, Gapstur SM, Folsom AR. Sugar, meat, and fat intake, and non-dietary risk factors for colon cancer incidence in Iowa women. Cancer Causes Control 1994; 5:38–52.

80. Wu-Williams AH, Lee M, Whittemore AS, Gallagher RP, Deng-Ao J, Lun Z, Xianghu W, Kun C, Jung D, Chengde L, Yao XJ, Paffenbarger RS Jr, Henderson BE. Reproductive factors and colorectal cancer risk among Chinese females. Cancer Res 1991; 51:2307–2311.

81. Peters RK, Pike MC, Chang WWL, Mack TM. Reproductive factors and colon cancers. Br J Cancer 1990; 61:741–748.

82. Davis FG, Furner SE, Persky V, Koch M. The influence of parity and exogenous female hormones on the risk of colorectal cancer. Int J Cancer 1989; 43:587–590.

83. Adami HO, Persson I, Hoover R, Schairer C, Bergkvist L. Risk of cancer in women receiving hormone replacement therapy. Int J Cancer 1989; 44:833–839.

84. Wu AH, Paganini-Hill A, Ross RK, Henderson BE. Alcohol, physical activity, and other risk factors for colorectal cancer: a prospective study. Br J Cancer 1987; 55:687–694.

85. Potter JD, McMichael AJ. Large bowel cancer in women in relation to reproductive and hormonal factors: a case-control study. J Natl Cancer Inst 1983; 71:703–709.

86. Weiss NS, Daling JR, Chow WH. Incidence of cancer of the large bowel in women in relation to reproductive and hormonal factors. J Natl Cancer Inst 1981; 67:57–60.

87. Fernandez E, La Vecchia C, Braga C, Talamini R, Negri E, Parazzini F, Franceschi S. Hormone replacement therapy and risk of colon rectal cancer. Cancer Epidemiol Biomarkers and Prev 1998; 7:329–333.

88. Franceschi S, La Vecchia C. Oral contraceptives and colon colorectal tumors; a review of epidemiologic studies. Contraception 1998; 58:335–343.

89. La Vecchia C, Ron E, Franceschi S, Dal Maso L, Mark SD, Chatenoud L, Braga C, Preston-Marton S, McTiernan A, Kolonel L, Mabuchi K, Jin F, Wingren G, Galanti MR, Hallquist A, Lund E, Lebi F, Linos D, Negri E. A pooled analysis of case-control studies of thyroid cancer. Cancer Causes Control; 1999; 10:156–166.

90. Writing group for the Women's Health Initiative Investigators. Risks and benefits of estrogen plus progestin in healthy postmenopausal women. Principal results from the Women's Health Initiative randomized controlled trial. JAMA 2002; 288:321–333.

5

Alternatives to Hormonal Replacement Therapy for Prevention of Osteoporosis

Richard Kremer and David Goltzman
McGill University and McGill University Health Centre, Montreal, Quebec, Canada

I. OVERVIEW

Osteoporosis is defined as a systemic skeletal disease characterized by low bone mass and microarchitecture deterioration of bone tissue, with a consequent increase in bone fragility and susceptibility to fractures [1]. According to this definition, both quantitative and qualitative factors contribute to the risk of bone fractures. Quantitatively, there is a significant reduction of the amount of bone and qualitatively, the trabecular struts are thinned and prone to perforation. It is estimated that 1 in 4 women over 50 years of age and 1 in 8 men over 50 years of age suffer from osteoporosis, and that 70% of hip fractures are the result of osteoporosis [2]. Furthermore, up to 20% of women who fracture a hip die in less than a year [3]. This burden of illness, which is estimated at more than 15 billion dollars per year in North America alone for acute and long term healthcare costs, is predicted to increase to 50 billion by the year 2040, vastly surpassing the cost of other chronic illnesses [4].

Following menopause, the spine is a key site of bone loss in women. This bone loss which occurs in the trabecular bone of vertebrae leads to multiple compression deformities with subsequent height loss and dorsal kyphosis [5] These vertebral deformities are permanent and may result in a decreased thoracic volume, compression of abdominal structures, back pain [6], and psychosocial impairment [7]. In addition to physical and functional impairments, prevalent vertebral deformities are associated with a 5-fold increased risk of developing another vertebral deformity and a 2.8-fold increased risk of hip fracture [8] There are a number of well-established risk factors for osteoporosis including genetic background; advanced age; White race; estrogen deficiency; drug therapy, such as corticosteroids; and lifestyle habits, such as inactivity and smoking [9,10].

II. DIAGNOSIS AND PATHOPHYSIOLOGY

Because osteoporosis is a slow process in the vast majority of patients, bone loss occurs long before the development of fractures. Consequently, bone mass measurement is the only objective tool to aid in the early diagnosis of this condition. Several methods have been developed for bone mass measurements, including dual energy x-ray absorptiometry (DXA), quantitative computed tomography (QCT) scan, and quantitative ultrasound (QUS) [11]. Because DXA provides high resolution, reproducibility, and fast scan times, it is the reference standard for bone mineral density (BMD) measurements [11,12]. Interpretation of BMD has recently been defined by the World Health Organization (WHO) based on T score values [13]. The T score expresses standard deviation differences from the peak bone mass of the young adult age group (20–35 years). Therefore, T score compares the BMD of a given subject with the expected maximum BMD (peak bone mass) adjusted for the sex and race. According to the WHO, subjects can be divided into four categories (see Table 1). Although there is no consensus for screening the population at large with BMD measurements, it is recommended when certain risk factors are identified, including: premature menopause (<45 years old), family history of osteoporosis (in first-degree relatives), previous fracture with minimal trauma (fragility fracture), low body weight, glucocorticoid therapy, malabsorption, anticonvulsant therapy, primary hyperparathyroidism, and chemotherapy

Table 1   WHO Interpretation of BMD Results

T score	Diagnosis
	Normal
	BMD less than 1.0 standard deviation (SD) below the T score[a]
−1	Osteopenia
	BMD 1.0 to 2.5 SD below the T score
−2.5	Osteoporosis
	BMD more than 2.5 SD below the T score
	Severe osteoporosis
	BMD more than 2.5 SD below the T score and the presence of one or more fragility fractures.

[a] T score is defined in comparison with the young adult reference range, whereas the Z score is defined in comparison with same-age, sex-matched population.

exposure. In addition to a low bone density, bone quality may also play an important role in the development of osteoporotic fractures, but is more complex to measure.

To understand current and future therapies of osteoporosis, it is important to examine briefly the bone remodeling cycle. The first step in this cycle is the creation of a resorption cavity by active osteoclasts (multinucleated bone resorbing cells). Following their activation, osteoclasts release hydrogen ions and enzymes through the ruffled border to degrade bone matrix. The attachment of osteoclasts to the bone matrix is mediated by adhesion molecules [14]. The second step is the formation stage whereby osteoblast (bone forming cells) migrate to the bone surface of the resorption pit and lay down new bone matrix. The final step is the resting phase in which quiescent osteoblasts line the bone surface. With age and especially after menopause, the rate of bone resorption tends to exceed the rate of bone formation, resulting in a slow decrease in bone mass [15]. This imbalance between bone formation and resorption can be detected by measuring biochemical markers of bone turnover in blood or urine (Table 2). Although bone turnover biochemical markers may predict fracture risk, they are primarily used to monitor treatment of osteoporosis because their change occurs more rapidly (within 3 months) than BMD (more than 1 year).

Table 2 Biochemical Markers of Bone Turnover

Bone resorption	Bone formation
Urine	Serum bone alkaline phosphatase
C- and N-telopeptides	Serum C- and N-propeptides of
Pyridinium crosslinks of collagen	type I collagen
Hydroxyproline	Serum osteocalcin
Galactosyl hydrolysine	
Serum	
C- and N-telopeptides	
Tartrate-resistant acid phosphatase	

III. MECHANISM OF ANTIRESORPTIVE AND ANABOLIC THERAPIES

The major goal of treating patients with osteoporosis is to decrease the risk of fracture. Numerous studies have shown a strong relationship between the reduction in risk of fractures and improvements in BMD [16,17]. On the basis of these studies, it is estimated that the risk of new vertebral fractures doubles for each standard deviation (SD) decrease in BMD. However, more recent clinical trials indicate that other factors may also be important, such as bone quality [18]. These studies suggest that bone strength may also be improved without significantly increasing bone mass in a substantial proportion of patients.

Current and future treatments of osteoporosis work by either inhibiting bone resorption (antiresorptive agents) or by stimulating bone formation (bone forming/anabolic agents). Other agents work by improving nutritional status, muscle mass, or by unknown mechanisms (Table 3). To better understand the current and future strategies to treat osteoporosis, it is important to briefly review some recent developments in bone biology, and in particular, the mechanism of osteoblastic and osteoclastic differentiation (Fig. 1). The precursors of these cells are found in the bone marrow. Osteoblasts originate from mesenchymal stem cells (MSCs) [19]. These pluripotent MSCs not only contribute to the generation and regeneration of bone, but also to the formation of adipose, cartilage, and muscle tissues [20]. Osteoclasts (bone resorbing cells) are large multinucleated cells derived from hematopoietic precur-

Table 3   Therapeutic Agents for Osteoporosis

Current treatments	Under investigation
Antiresorptive	Antiresorptive
Estrogens with or without progestins	New SERMs
Selective estrogen receptor modulators	New bisphosphonates
(SERMs)	Ibandronate
Raloxifene (Evista®)	Zoledronate (Zometa®)
Tamoxifen	
Bisphosphonates	
Alendronate (Fosamax®)	
Residronate (Actonel®)	
Etidronate (Didrocal®)	
Nasal calcitonin (Miacalcin®)	
Anabolic	
Fluoride	Anabolic
Parathyroid hormone [1–34] (Forteo®)	Parathyroid hormone and
Others	parathyroid hormone re-
Calcium plus vitamin D	lated peptide analogs
1,25 dihydroxyvitamin D	Growth hormone
Anabolic steroids	

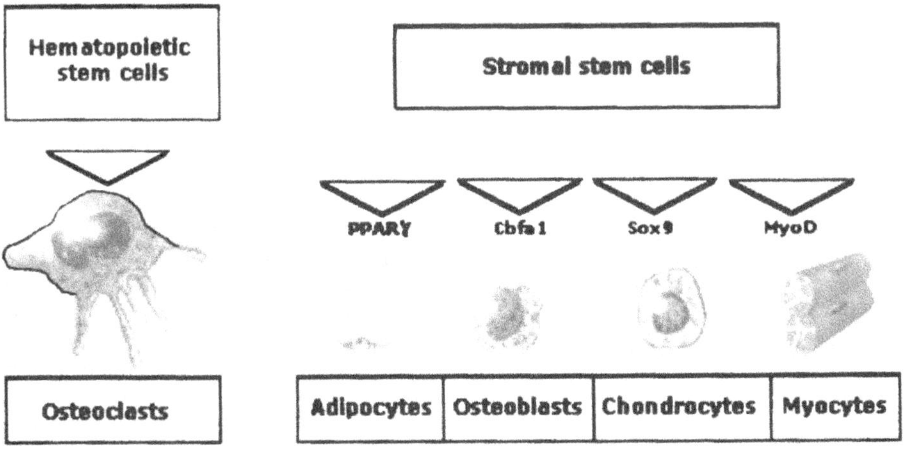

Figure 1   Schematic representation of bone marrow stem cell lineages and genes involved in differentiation of stromal stem cells.

sors of the monocyte macrophage lineage [21]. Major advances have
been made in the last several years to unravel the key factors involved
in osteoblast and osteoclast differentiation. In addition, there is mount-
ing evidence that regulation of adipogenesis within the bone marrow
may play an important role in the development of osteoporosis, because
accumulation of fat cells occurs at the expense of bone formation
[22,23]. Because interconversion between adipocytes and osteoblasts
is possible in vitro [24], it is tempting to speculate that conversion of
osteoblasts to adipocytes within the bone marrow may contribute to
osteoporosis. It also opens the possibility that this ability to change
phenotype of MSCs may be manipulated pharmacologically. A number
of key genes have recently been identified that govern these differentiation pathways. Osteoblast specific factor 2/core binding factor (*Cbfal*)
is required for commitment of MSCs to the osteoblast lineage [25,26].
Peroxisome proliferation activated receptor γ (*PPARγ*) controls adipocyte differentiation [27], whereas *Sox 9* and *Myo D* control chondrocyte
and myocyte differentiation, respectively [28,29]. A number of factors
are potent stimulators of bone turnover (Table 4) [30] and are often
produced by bone cells or cells in the bone microenvironment, acting
in an autocrine–paracrine fashion. The most important systemic factor
regulating bone turnover is parathyroid hormone (PTH), which has a
dual effect on bone mediated by the osteoblast. PTH binds a PTH receptor on the surface of osteoblastic cells and via these cells induces
both bone formation and resorption. PTH effect on bone resorption is
indirect and is mediated by the recently characterized tumor necrosis
factor-like molecule receptor activation of NF-kB (RANK) ligand

Table 4 Stimulators of Bone Turnover

Bone resorption	Bone formation
Epidermal growth factor (EGF)	Bone morphogenetic proteins
Fibroblast growth factors (FGFs)	(BMPs)
Granulocyte/macrophage colony	Fibroblast growth factors (FGFs)
stimulating factor (GM-CSF)	Insulin-like growth factors (IGFs)
Interleukins (ILs)	Platelet-derived growth factors
Osteoprotegerin Ligand (OPGL)	(PDGFs)
Tumor necrosis factors (TNFs)	Transforming growth factor β
	(TGFβ)

(RANKL), also called osteoclast differentiation factor (ODF) or osteo-protegerin ligand (OPGL) [31]. This factor is expressed at the surface of the osteoblast following PTH stimulation and then binds to its cognate receptor, RANK, on the osteoclast to stimulate osteoclastic activity in response to PTH [32]. A soluble decoy receptor called osteoprotegerin (OPG) can also be produced by osteoblastic stromal cells and binds RANKL, blocking its binding to receptor sites on osteoclasts [33]. Pharmacological manipulation of the RANKL/OPG system may therefore be beneficial in improving bone mass and treating osteoporosis [33,34].

As indicated earlier, the vast majority of currently approved therapies for osteoporosis are aimed at inhibiting osteoclastic bone resorption (Table 3). Although the mechanism whereby estrogens inhibit bone resorption is unclear, major advances have been made in elucidating the mechanism of action of bisphosphonates (BPs) (Fig. 2). These analogs of pyrophosphate share a common P–C–P backbone with different side chains attached to the central carbon atom. The earlier and less potent version of BPs, such as etidronate and clodronate, differ from the newer, most potent BPs (alendronate, ibandronate, olpadronate, pamidronate, risedronate, and zoledronate) by a shorter carbon-based side chain and the absence of a nitrogen atom in the side chain. They also differ in their mechanism of action. Non-amino-bisphosphonates such as etidronate and clodronate have been shown to be metabolized into adenosine triphosphate (ATP) analogs, which results in the induction of necrosis and apoptosis of target cells [35]. In contrast, amino-bisphosphonates act by inhibiting the cholesterol biosynthetic pathway like the statins, which are potent inhibitors of 3-hydroxy-3-methylglutaryl coenzyme A (HMG-CoA) reductase. Amino-bisphosphonates inhibit cholesterol synthesis downstream of HMG-CoA reductase at an enzyme called farnesyldiphosphate (FPP) synthase [36,37] (Fig. 2). This enzyme inhibition results in a protein–lipid modification called isoprenylation. The functional consequences of inhibition of protein prenylation by BPs include loss of ruffled border (function) and loss of survival (apoptosis) of osteoclasts [38].

On the basis of the elucidation of the mechanisms of bone turnover, a number of additional treatment options are now emerging that are based on decreasing osteoclastogenesis or on increasing osteoblastogenesis (Table 5).

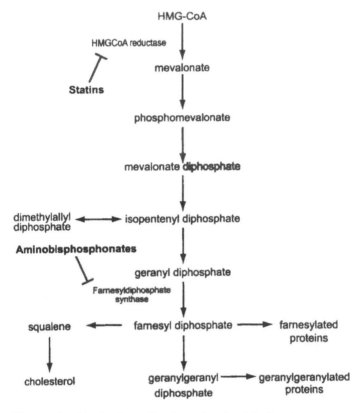

Figure 2   Mechanism of action of amino-bisphosphonates.

Table 5   Emerging Therapies for Osteoporosis

Inhibitors of osteoclastogenesis	Stimulators of osteoblastogenesis
Osteoprotegerin (OPG)	Growth factors: IGFs, TGFβ,
Proton (H⁺) pump inhibitors	BMPs, etc.
Inhibitors of enzymes released by active osteoclasts	Intracellular gene targets: Cbfa1 or Cbfa1 regulators
Inhibitors of adhesion molecules	
Inhibitors of bone resorbing cyto-kines (GM-CSF, IL, TNFs, etc.)	

IV. CURRENT AND FUTURE THERAPIES
OF OSTEOPOROSIS

A number of pharmacological agents are now available based on the results of large placebo-controlled randomized clinical trials. However, there is no clear consensus on who should be treated and which agent should be preferred. In addition to pharmacological agents, a number of measures can help reduce fracture risk. Lifestyle changes such as stopping smoking, discontinuing heavy alcohol intake, and engaging in weight-bearing exercises may reduce fracture risk by improving muscle strength and reducing the risk of falling [9,39]. In elderly people measures have been advocated such as restricting the use of sedative medications to prevent falls and encouraging the use of "hip protectors" to decrease hip fractures. Calcium and vitamin D supplements are also part of the routine regimen in the treatment or prevention of osteoporosis. A number of studies indicate that both calcium and vitamin D absorption by the gut [40,41] and vitamin D production by the skin [42] decrease with age. Furthermore, combined therapy with calcium and vitamin D has been shown to reduce rates of nonvertebral fractures in the elderly [43,44]. Consequently, patients should have sufficient daily intake of calcium (1000 mg daily of elemental calcium for premenopausal women and 1500 mg for postmenopausal women) and vitamin D (400–800 IU per day) through either diet or supplements [45]. We will review the evidence for pharmacotherapy based on published clinical trials and will attempt to compare the efficacy of the therapies (Table 6).

A. Antiresorptive Therapies

The vast majority of currently approved therapies for either prevention or treatment of osteoporosis act by inhibiting bone resorption. Estrogen replacement therapy (ERT) and selective estrogen receptor modulators (SERMs) fall into this category but will not be discussed in detail in this chapter. ERT has long been approved for the prevention and treatment of postmenopausal osteoporosis based primarily on epidemiologic studies [46]. These studies indicated a reduction of fracture risk at the hip and forearm, but could not predict effects on vertebral fractures.

Table 6 Summary of Results of the Large Randomized Double-Blind Placebo-Controlled Trials

	PROOF (Miacalcin)®	MORE (Evista)®	FIT (Fosamax)® First arm	VERT (Residronate)®
Follow-up Inclusion criteria	5-year study >1 and ≤5 VFx	3-year study BMD T score < −2.5 or existing VFx	3-year study ≥1 VFx BMD T score ≤ −1.6	3-year study ≥1 VFx BMD T score ≤ −2
No. of patients (with VF at baseline)	990 of 1255 (79%)	2641 of 6828 (34%)	2027 of 2027 (100%)	1284 of 2458 (52%)
Dosage	Miacalcin 100 IU Miacalcin 200 IU Miacalcin 400 IU	Evista 60 mg Evista 120 mg	Fosamax 5 mg (2 years) 10 mg (third year)	Residronate 2.5 mg (lasted 1 year) Residronate 5 mg
Calcium (Ca) + vitamin D (D)	1000 mg Ca + 400 IU D	500 mg Ca + 400 IU D	*500 mg Ca + 250 IU D	1000 mg Ca + 500 IU D
Primary endpoint NVF risk RR (95% CI)	Reduction in NVFx 0.64 (0.43–0.96) $P = 0.03$	Reduction in NVFx 0.70 (0.58–0.86) 60 mg 0.50 (0.39–0.63) 120 mg	Reduction in NVFx 0.53 (0.41–0.68) $P < 0.001$	Reduction in NVFx 0.59 (0.43–0.81) $P = 0.003$
Risk reduction	36%	30% & 50%, respectively	47%	41%

NNT	10	16 (60mg) 10 (120 mg)	14	N/A
MVF (>2) risk reduction	45%	61%	90%	77%
Hip Fx risk: RR (95% CI)	0.52 (0.17–1.56) P = NS	1.1 (0.64–1.99) P = NS	0.49 (0.23–0.99) P = 0.047	0.70 (0.6–0.9)[a] p = 0.02
Risk reduction	48%	10% (increased risk)	51%	30%
Wrist Fx risk: RR (95% CI)	0.75 (0.36–1.56) P = N	0.88 (0.68–1.14) P = NS	0.52 (0.31–0.87) p = 0.013	N/A
Risk reduction	25%	12%	48%	
Non-VFx: RR (95% CI)	P = NS	P = NS	0.64 (0.5–0.82) P = 0.02	0.6 (0.39–.094) P = 0.02
Risk reduction			36%	39%

LS = lumbar spine; BMD = bone mineral density; RR = relative risk; NS = non-significant; NNT = number needed to treat (represents how many patients need to be treated to prevent one new vertebral fracture); VFx = vertebral fracture; NVFx = new vertebral fracture; MVFx = multiple vertebral fractures; Fx-fracture.

[a] Not from VERT data but from the Hip Intervention Program Study Group.

Furthermore, acceptance and compliance with long-term ERT is a major problem because only one-third of postmenopausal women are willing to accept it [9] and more than 40% are not compliant at 1 year. To complicate this issue, a recent large placebo-controlled trial indicated no reduction of hip or clinical fractures in postmenopausal women treated with ERT as compared to placebo [47]. Currently in the United States, a large prospective randomized trial sponsored by the National Institutes of Health (NIH) is examining the effect of estrogen on bone, heart, and breast. SERMs are a new class of agents with estrogenic-blocking actions at the breast but estrogenic-positive actions on bone and lipids. Currently available agents include raloxifene and tamoxifen. Raloxifene has the advantage over tamoxifen of not inducing uterine stimulation or uterine cancer. In a large prospective randomized trial of more than 7000 women (Multiple Outcomes of Raloxifene Evaluation [MORE]), raloxifene treatment for 3 years significantly reduced the risk of vertebral fractures by 30% in the bone group and by 50% in the 120-mg group in patients with preexisting vertebral fractures, but had no effect on nonvertebral or hip fractures [48]. Notably, these positive effects on vertebral fracture reduction occurred despite modest increase in BMD (1–3%). In addition, raloxifene may reduce breast cancer risk by more than 60%.

Bisphosphonate Therapies

Cyclical intermittent Etidronate (90-day dosage cycle with 14 days of etidronate followed by 76 days of elemental calcium) was the first BP to be approved in Europe and Canada for use in postmenopausal osteoporosis. Etidronate produces inhibition of mineralization of the bone matrix (osteomalacia) when administered continuously, a side effect which can be reduced by using an intermittent cyclical regimen. A placebo-controlled study indicated that this regimen increased bone density by an average of 5% and reduced the risk of vertebral fractures by about 50% [49], but only in patients with advanced disease (with three or more prevalent vertebral fractures). This trial was then extended to 7 years and patients were categorized by their total years of cumulative etidronate therapy. This study indicates a strong inverse correlation between years of therapy and the risk of vertebral fractures [50].

The most unambiguous evidence for the efficacy of BP in fracture prevention of postmenopausal osteoporosis was first provided by studies with the amino-bisphosphonate alendronate. In the first clinical trial, continuous alendronate treatment for 3 years in 994 women with postmenopausal osteoporosis caused a significant increase in BMD at all skeletal sites, the effect being most important at the spine ($\cong 8\%$), and a significant reduction in the risk of new vertebral fractures by approximately 50% [51]. The effect of alendronate on vertebral and nonvertebral fractures was further assessed in 2027 women with preexisting vertebral fractures (Fracture Intervential Trial [FIT]), which indicated that alendronate treatment for 3 years significantly reduced new vertebral fractures but also fractures at the hip and wrist by approximately 50% (52). Furthermore, alendronate reduced the risk of multiple new vertebral fractures (>1) by more than 90%. FIT also analyzed a subgroup of 4432 postmenopausal women with low BMD but no prevalent vertebral fractures [53]. Alendronate reduced the risk of vertebral fractures and clinical fractures in women whose T scores were ≤ -2.5, but did not offer a fracture benefit to women with higher baseline BMD (T score of -1.6 to -2.5).

As with any BP, alendronate is poorly absorbed when taken orally ($<1\%$). Furthermore, oral bioavailability is further reduced by prior food intake and concomitant administration of calcium-containing food or supplements. Consequently, alendronate should be administered after an overnight fast, at least 30 min before breakfast with water only. Certain precautions such as not reclining after ingesting the medication should be taken with alendronate therapy, because gastrointestinal adverse events have been reported in postmarketing studies including esophagitis, and gastric and duodenal ulcers. Recently, a clinical trial was completed in 1258 women with postmenopausal osteoporosis using alendronate 70 mg once weekly that showed comparable efficacy to the 10 mg daily regimen based on changes in BMD and biochemical markers. Furthermore, the incidence of esophageal and gastroduodenal adverse experiences tended to be lower when administered once weekly, making this regimen more convenient and possibly safer than the daily regimen [54].

Risedronate is the most recent BP to be approved for the treatment of postmenopausal osteoporosis. In a large study involving 2458 postmenopausal women with a median of two prevalent vertebral fractures

(Vertebral Efficacy with Residronate Therapy [VERT]), residronate treatment increased lumbar spine BMD by 7.1% and femoral neck BMD by 2.1%, and reduced both vertebral and nonvertebral fractures by approximately 40% [55]. Risedronate was also assessed in a large trial involving over 8000 postmenopausal women with hip fracture as the primary end point [56]. This study concluded that residronate significantly reduced the risk of hip fracture by 40% in women with confirmed osteoporosis, but not in women selected primarily on the basis of risk factors other than low BMD. There were no apparent gastrointestinal side effects in the residronate group as compared to placebo, which may prove to be an advantage.

Calcitonin

Calcitonin is a peptide hormone composed of a chain of 32 amino acids and has been shown to inhibit osteoclastic activity after binding to specific receptors on these cells. Salmon calcitonin is the most potent and longest acting species of calcitonin, even in humans, and its effect has been evaluated in a 5-year prospective randomized trial involving over 1200 women (Prevent Recurrence of Osteoporotic Fractures [PROOF]). Salmon calcitonin nasal spray was used in a 100-, 200- or 400-IU daily regimen with patients with one to five prevalent vertebral fractures. All patients received 1000 mg of elemental calcium and 400 IU vitamin D daily. At 5 years, a modest increase in BMD (1–1.5%) was observed in all treatment groups and the risk of developing new vertebral fractures was significantly reduced by 36% in patients receiving 200 IU salmon–calcitonin nasal spray compared to placebo. However, neither the lower (100 IU) nor the higher (400 IU) doses had an effect [57]. The lack of a dose response and the relatively low number of patients completing the study (378 of 1255) weakened the results of this trial. On the other hand, salmon calcitonin nasal spray is generally well tolerated with few adverse events except for occasional rhinitis. Furthermore, the analgesic effect of calcitonin, reported in earlier studies, may be an added benefit of this agent [58].

Combined Antiresorptive Therapies

In a 4-year study, 72 postmenopausal osteoporotic women with at least one vertebral fracture were randomized to either hormone replacement therapy (HRT), intermittent cyclical etidronate, HRT and etidronate, or placebo. This study demonstrated a significant additive effect of HRT and etidronate on both hip and spinal BMD [59]. Another study involving 428 postmenopausal osteoporotic women examined the effect of HRT in combination with alendronate. After 12 months of therapy, alendronate plus HRT produced a signficantly higher increase in BMD when compared to HRT alone [60]. However, none of these trials was powered for assessing fracture risk, and therefore further data are needed to evaluate combination therapy in the treatment of postmenopausal osteoporosis.

B. Anabolic Therapies

Treatment strategies for osteoporosis can be divided into those that decrease bone resorption and those that increase bone formation. Antiresorptive drugs have an indirect and temporary effect on bone mass as bone resporption decreases rapidly during the first 1–2 years of treatment, resulting in "filling in" of resorption spaces. The overall increase in bone mass is relatively moderate (5–10%) and is often not sufficient to increase BMD over and above the low level at which fractures may be occurring. Thus, these therapies have been shown at best to reduce fracture risk by 50%. Bone-forming agents are therefore needed to increase bone mass sufficiently to further reduce or even completely eliminate the risk of fracture. In theory these could be the agents of choice given alone or in combination with anti-resorptive agents for the treatment of osteoporosis.

Fluoride

Sodium fluoride (NaF) has been known to stimulate bone formation for many years, but its efficacy in osteoporosis remains controversial. All studies show a significant increase in spinal BMD on the order of 6% [61,62], but the effect of NaF on fracture risk may be dependent on the dosage used. There is concern that fluoride may indeed increase the risk of nonvertebral fractures, and in particular, hip fracture. Consequently, there may be discordance between the increase in mineral density and the mechanical strength of bone newly formed under the influence of fluoride.

Table 7 Clinical studies with PTH Analogs

Analog	Placebo	Combination	Patients	Duration	BMD Change
hPTH (1–34)[a] 500 U sc/day	No	Estrogens	Osteoporosis (10 females and 1 male) $n = 12$	12 months	↑50% at LS
hPTH (1–34)[b] 500 U sc/day	No	1,25(OH)$_2$D$_3$ (0.25 µg/day)	PMO $n = 15$	12–24 months	↑12% at LS
hPTH(1–34)[c] 500 U sc/day (100 µg)	No	1,25(OH)$_2$D$_3$ (0.25 µg/day)	Males with OP $n = 8$	12 months	↑198% at LS
hPTH (1–34)[d] 40 µg sc/day	Yes	Nafarelin (GHRH analog)	Premenopausal women with induced hypogonadism $n = 40$	6 months	↑3.5% at LS

Treatment		Concomitant	Population	Duration	Results
hPTH (1–34)[e] 800 U sc/day	Yes	Calcitonin (CT) 75 U/day	PMO $n = 30$	24 months	↑10.2% at LS (PTH alone) ↑7.9% at LS (PTH + CT)
hPTH (1–38)[f] 400 U sc/day (25 µg)	Yes	Estrogens	PMO $n = 34$	12 months	↑13% at LS ↑2.7% at hip
hPTH (1–34)[g] 20 or 40 µg sc/day	Yes	No	PMO $n = 1637$	21 months	↑9% at LS (20 µg) ↑13% at LS (40 µg) ↑3% at hip (20 µg) ↑6% at hip (40 µg)

PMO = postmenopausal osteoporosis; OP = osteoporosis; LS = lumbar spine; PTH = parathyroid hormone; CT = calcitonin; sc = subcutaneous.

[a] Source: Ref. 71.
[b] Source: Ref. 72.
[c] Source: Ref. 73.
[d] Source: Ref. 74.
[e] Source: Ref. 75.
[f] Source: Ref. 76.
[g] Source: Ref. 77.

Growth Hormone

A number of in vitro and animal studies indicate that growth hormone (GH) has an anabolic effect on bone [63,64]. Growth hormone has subsequently been given to postmenopausal women alone or in combination with antiresorptive medications. The increase in BMD was moderate at both spine and hip (2–3%) [65], and there are no reports yet on fracture reduction in large clinical trials.

Parathyroid Hormone

The most exciting development in anabolic therapy comes from studies using derivatives of the natural peptide parathyroid hormone (PTH). Parathyroid hormone is an 84-amino acid peptide produced by the parathyroid glands, which together with 1,25-dihydroxyvitamin D is a major regulator of calcium homeostasis [66]. When PTH is administered exogenously, the net effect on bone turnover depends on its mode of delivery. A continuous infusion of PTH results in a net increase in bone resorption and decreased bone mass, whereas daily single injections result in a net increase in bone formation with increased bone mass [67,68] This anabolic effect of PTH is proportional to the dose and more pronounced in trabecular than cortical bone [69], but its mechanism is poorly understood. Animal studies have shown that bone quality is preserved [70]. Several studies have been undertaken in osteoporotic patients with various forms of human (h)PTH alone or in combination with antiresorptive agents [71–76] (Table 7). BMD increased rapidly even in the presence of concommittant antiresorptive therapy [76]. However, none of these earlier studies were powered to detect a reduction in fracture rate. Recently a large, multicenter, double-blind, randomized clinical trial addressed this question in 1637 postmenopausal women with one or more prevalent vertebral fractures. Patients were given either placebo, 20 μg, or 40 μg of recombinant hPTH [1–34] by once daily self-injection subcutaneously for up to 2 years. All patients received 1000 mg of elemental calcium/day with 400–1200 IU of vitamin D. This study concluded that hPTH [1–34] decreased the risk of new vertebral fractures by more than 65% and decreased the risk of nontraumatic, nonvertebral fractures by 54%. The increase in BMD was also substantial, with a 9–13% increase at the lumbar spine and 3–6% increase at the femoral neck in less than 2 years. Only minor side effects were noted, including nausea, headaches, and leg cramps. Transient and minor increase in circulating serum calcium levels were noted [77]. On the basis of these results, (h)PTH [1–34] has recently been approved for the treatment of postmenopausal osteoporosis.

V. SUMMARY

Prevention and treatment of postmenopausal osteoporosis involves a multifold approach. It involves weight-bearing exercise [78,79], avoidance of tobacco and heavy alcohol consumption, and adequate calcium and vitamin D intake, especially in the elderly where subclinical vitamin D deficiency is common. The pharmacological approach and the utility of various agents to reduce the risk of hip and spinal fractures is best addressed using BMD measurements according to the National Osteoporosis Foundation (NOF) guidelines [2]. According to these guidelines, postmenopausal women with a T score ≤ -2 in the absence of other risk factors and ≤ -1.5 in the presence of other risk factors should be considered for pharmacological treatment. In addition, all women above age 70 years, especially those with a history of clinical fracture, should be considered. Although overall fracture risk can be predicted from BMD measurement at the lumbar spine, hip fracture risk is best predicted by BMD measurement at the proximal femur. It is not generally recommended to start a pharmacological agent before menopause unless some additional factor(s) is present which can seriously and rapidly affect bone loss, such as the use of glucocorticoids. Addition of a pharmacological agent should be monitored with BMD measurements to assess treatment response and ensure patient compliance by active involvement in the overall management. BMD changes over time are often moderate and may vary considerably between patients and with the pharmacological agent employed. However, it should be clear to the patient that even a small increment in BMD will result in a very significant reduction of fracture risk. Assessment of BMD changes can also be affected by intra-instrument variability and the lack of standardization between different bone densitometers. It is therefore best to perform BMD testing with the same instrument to minimize variability and to interpret results after several annual measurements.

In the absence of direct head-to-head comparisons between drugs in large clinical trials, the choice of the pharmacological agent rests mainly on risk assessment, goals of therapy, and patient preference. Apart from ERT–HRT and raloxifene, which target several organs, other agents are bone specific. Intranasal salmon calcitonin reduces vertebral fracture risk, but has no effect on hip and other fractures. The newer bisphosphonates (alendronate and residronate) offer a good alternative because they have been shown to reduce fracture risk at both the spine and hip with minimal side effects. Finally, an important addition to this therapeutic armamentarium comes from the recent approval of the anabolic agent PTH. The rapid and impressive effect of PTH on both BMD increase and fracture reduction at hip and spine provides an additional tool in our therapeutic armamentarium.

Ongoing and future clinical trials should help us to rationalize the use of antiresorptive and anabolic agents given alone or in combination, not only in postmenopausal osteoporosis, but also in all forms of osteoporosis in both men and women.

ACKNOWLEDGMENTS

We thank Mike Macoritto for preparation of figures, and Carmen Ferrara for preparation of the manuscript.

REFERENCES

1. European Foundation Osteoporosis and the National Osteoporosis Foundation. Consensus development statement: who are candidates for prevention and treatment for osteoporosis? Osteoporos Int 1997; 7:1–6.
2. Physician's guide to prevention and treatment of osteoporosis. Washington DC: National Osteoporosis Foundation, 1998.
3. Hodgson SF, Johnston CC Jr. For the Osteoporosis Task Force. AACE clinical practice guidelines for the prevention and treatment of postmenopausal osteoporosis. Endocr Pract 1996; 1:155–171.

4. Miller PD. Management of osteoporosis. Adv Int Med 1999; 44:175–207.
5. Riggs BL. Overview of osteoporosis. West J Med 1991; 154:63–77.
6. Cummings SR, Kelsey JL, Nevitt MC, O'Dowd KJ. Epidemiology of osteoporosis and osteoporotic fractures. Epidermiol Rev 1985; 7:178–208.
7. Lyles KW, Gold DT, Shipp KM, Pieper CF. Martinez S. Mulhausen PL. Association of osteoporotic vertebral compression fractures with impaired functional status. Am J Med 1993; 94:595–601.
8. Black DM, Arden NK, Palermo L. Pearson J. Cummings SR. Prevalent vertebral deformities predict hip fractures and new vertebral deformities but not wrist fractures. J Bone Miner Res 1999; 14:821–828.
9. Consensus Development Conference. Diagnosis, prophylaxis, and treatment of osteoporosis. Am J Med 1993; 94:646–650.
10. Cummings SR, Nevitt MC, Browner WS, Stone K. Fox KM. Ensrud KE. Cauley J. Black D, Vogt TM. Risk factors for hip fracture in white women. N Engl J Med 1995; 332:767–773.
11. Genant HK, Engelke K, Fuerst T, Gluer CC, Grampp S, Harris ST, Jergas M, Lang T, Lu Y, Majumdar S, Mathur A, Takada M. Noninvasive assessment of bone mineral and structure: state of the art. J Bone Miner Res 1996; 11:707–730.
12. Notelovitz M. Osteoporosis: screening, prevention and management. Fertil Steril 1993; 59:707–725.
13. WHO Technical Report Series 843. Assessment of fracture risk and its application to screening for post-menopausal osteoporosis. Geneva: World Health Organization, 1994.
14. Horton MA, Davies J. Perspectives: adhesion receptors in bone. J Bone Miner Res 1989; 4:803–807.
15. Eastell R. Treatment of post menopausal osteoporosis. N Engl J Med 1998; 338:736–746.
16. Wasnich R. Bone mass measurement: prediction of risk. Am J Med 1993; 95: 65–105.
17. Millard PS, Rosen CJ, Johnson KH. Osteoporotic vertebral fractures in post-menopausal women. Am Fam Physician 1997; 55:1315–1322.
18. Dempster DW. The bone quality concept : relationships between bone remodeling, structure and integrity. Osteoporos Int 1998; 8(suppl 3): 137–139.
19. Owen ME. Lineage of osteogenic cells and their relationship to the stromal system. In: Peck WE, ed. Bone and Mineral Research. Vol 3. Amsterdam: Elsevier, 1985: 1–25.

20. Kuznetsov SA, Krebsbach PH, Satomura K, Kerr J, Riminucci M, Benayahu D, Robey PG. Single-colony derived strains of human marrow stromal fibroblasts form bone after transplantation in vivo. J Bone Miner Res 1997; 12:1335–1347.

21. Suda T, Takahashi N, Martin TJ. Modulation of osteoclast differentiation. Endocr Rev 1992; 13:66–80.

22. Jilka R, Weinstein RS, Takahashi K, Parfitt AM, Manolagas SC. Linkage of decreased bone mass with impaired osteoblastogenesis in a murine model of accelerated senescence. J Clin Invest 1996; 97:1732–1740.

23. Lecka-Czernik B, Gubrij I, Moerman EJ, Kajkenova O, Lipschitz DA, Manolagas SC, Jilka RL. Inhibition of Osf2/Cbfa1 expression and terminal osteoblast differentiation by PPARgamma2. J Cell Biochem 1999; 74:357–371.

24. Diascro DD, Vogel RL, Johnson TE, Witherup KM, Pitzenberger SM, Rutledge SJ, Prescott DJ, Rodan GA, Schmidt A. High fatty acid content in rabbit serum is responsible for the differentiation of osteoblasts into adipocyte-like cells. J Bone Min Res 1998; 13:96–106.

25. Komori T, Yagi H, Nomura S, Yamaguchi A, Sasaki K, Deguchi K, Shimizu Y, Bronson RT, Gao YH, Inada M, Sato M, Okamoto R, Kitamura Y, Yoshiki S, Kishimoto T. Targeted disruption of Cbfa1 results in a complete lack of bone formation owing to maturational arrest of osteoblasts. Cell 1997; 89:755–764.

26. Ducy P, Zhang R, Geoffroy V, Ridall AL, Karsenty G. Osf2/Cbfa1: a transcriptional activator of osteoblast differentiation. Cell 1997; 89:747–754.

27. Shao D, Lazar MA. Peroxisone proliferator activated receptor γ CCAAT/Enhancer binding protein α, and cell cycle status regulate the commitment to adipocyte differentiation. J Biol Chem 1997; 772: 21473–21478.

28. Lefevre V, Huang W, Harley VR, Goodfellow PN, de Crombrugghe B. Sox 9 is a potent activator of the chondrocyte-specific enhancer of the pro-alpha (II) collagen gene. Mol Cell Biol 1997; 17:2336–2346.

29. Pittenger MF, Mackay AM, Beck SC, Jaiswal RK, Douglas R, Mosca JD, Moorman MA, Simonette DW, Craig S, Marshak DR. Multilineage potential of adult mesenchymal stem cells. Science 1999; 284:143–147.

30. Manolagas SC, Jilka RL. Bone marrow, cytokines, and bone remodelling. N Engl J Med 1995; 332:305–311.

31. Lacey DL, Timms E, Tan HL, Kelley MJ, Dunstan CR, Burgess T, Elliott R, Colombero A, Elliott G, Scully S, Hsu H, Sullivan J, Hawkins N, Davy E, Capparelli C, Eli A, Qian YX, Kaufman S, Sarosi I, Shalhoub

V, Senaldi G, Guo J, Delaney J, Boyle WJ. Osteoprotegerin ligand is a cytokine that regulates osteoclast differentiation and activation. Cell 1998; 93:165–176.

32. Horwood NJ, Elliott J, Martin TJ, Gillespie MT. Osteotropic agents regulate the expression of osteoclast differentiation factor and osteoprotegerin in osteoblastic stromal cells. Endocrinology 1998; 139:4743–4746.

33. Simonet WS, Lacey DL, Dunstan CR, Kelley M, Chang MS, Luthy R, Nguyen HQ, Wooden S, Bennett L, Bonne T, Shimamoto G, DeRose M, Elliott R, Colombero A, Tan H-L, Trail G, Sullivan J, Davy E, Bucay N, Renshaw-Gegg L, Hughes TM, Hill D, Pattison W, Campbell P, Sander S, Van G, Tarplay J, Derby P, Lee R, Program AE, Boyle WJ. Osteoprotegerins: a novel secreted protein involved in the regulation of bone density cell. Cell 1997; 89:309–319.

34. Kong YY, Yoshida H, Sarosi I, Tan HL, Timms E, Caparelli C, Morony S, Santos AJO, Van G, Itie A, Khoo W, Wakeham A, Dunstan CR, Lacey DL, Mak TW, Boyle WJ, Penninger JM. OPGL is a key regulator of osteoclastogenesis, lymphocyte development and lymph node organogenesis. Nature 1999; 397:315–323.

35. Frith JC, Mönkkönen J, Blackburn GM, Russell RGG, Rogers MJ. Clodronate and liposome-encapsulated clodronate are metabolised to a toxic ATP analog, adenosine 5' triphosphate, by mammalian cells in vitro. J Bone Miner Res 1997; 12:1358–1367.

36. Luckman SP, Hughes DE, Coxon FP, Russell RGG and Rogers MJ. Nitrogen-containing bisphosphonates inhibit the mevalonate pathway and prevent post-translational prenylation of GTP binding proteins, including Ras. J Bone Miner Res 1998; 13: 581–589.

37. Fisher JE, Rogers MJ, Halasy JM, Luckman SP, Hughes DE, Masavachia PJ, Wesolowski J, Russell RGG, Rodan GA, Reszka AA. Alendronate mechanism of action. Geranylgeraniol, an intermediate in the mevalonate pathway prevents inhibition of osteoclast formation, some resorption and kinase activation in vitro. Proc Natl Acad Sci USA 1999; 96:133–138.

38. Ebetino FH, Francis MD, Rogers MJ, Russell RGG. Mechanisms of action of Etidronate and other bisphosphonates. Rev Contemp Pharmacother 1998; 9:233–243.

39. Lindsay R. Prevention and treatment of osteoporosis. Lancet 1993; 341: 801–805.

40. Bullamore JR, Wilkinson R, Gallagher JC, Nordin BEC, & Marshall DH. Effect of age on calcium absorption. Lancet 1970; ii:537.

41. Barragry JM, Franch MW, Corless D. Intestinal cholecalciferol absorption in the elderly and in younger adult. Clin Sci Mol Med 1978; 55: 213–220.

42. McLaughlin J, Holick MF. Aging decreases the capacity of human skin to produce vitamin D_3. J Clin Invest 1985; 76:1536–1538.

43. Dawson-Hughes B, Harris S, Krall E, Dallal GE. Effect of calcium and vitamin D supplementation on bone density in men and women 65 years of age or older. N Engl J Med 1997; 337:670–676.

44. Chapuy MC, Arlot ME, Duboeuf F, Brun J, Crouzet B, Arnaud S, Delmas PD, Meunier PJ. Vitamin D_3 and calcium to prevent hip fractures in elderly women. N Engl J Med 1992; 327:1637–1642.

45. NIH Consensus Development Panel on Optimal Calcium Intake: optimal calcium intake. JAMA 1994; 272:1942–1946.

46. Krel DP, Felson DT, Anderson JJ et al. Hip fracture and the use of estrogens in post-menopausal women. The Framingham Study. N Engl J Med 1987; 317:1169–1174.

47. Hulley S, Grady D, Bush T, Furberg C, Herrington D, Riggs B, Vittinghoff E. Randomized trial of estrogen plus progestin for secondary prevention of coronary heart disease in postmenopausal women. Heart and Estrogen/progestin Replacement Study (HERS) Research Group. JAMA 1998; 280:605-613.

48. Ettinger B, Black DM, Mitlak BH, Knickerbocker RK, Nickelsen T, Genant HK, Christiansen C, Delmas PD, Zanchetta JR, Stakkestad J, Gluer CC, Krueger K, Cohen FJ, Eckert S, Ensrud KE, Avioli LV, Lips P, Cummings SR. Reduction of vertebral fracture risk in postmenopausal women with osteoporosis treated with raloxifene: results from a 3-year randomized clinical trial. Multiple Outcomes of Raloxifene Evaluation (MORE) Investigators. JAMA 1999; 282:637–645.

49. Harris ST, Watts NB, Jackson RD, Genant HK, Wasnich RD, Ross P, Miller PD, Licata AA, Chesnut CH 3rd. Four year study of intermittent cyclic etidronate treatment of post-menopausal osteoporosis: three years of blinded therapy followed by one year of open therapy. Am J Med 1993; 95:557–567.

50. Miller PD, Watts NB, Licata AA, Harris ST, Genant HK, Wasnich RD, Ross PD, Jackson RD, Hoseyni MS, Schoenfeld SL, Valent DJ, Chesnut CH III. Cyclical etidronate in the treatment of post-menopausal osteoporosis: Efficacy and safety after seven years of treatment. Am J Med 1997; 103:468–476.

51. Lieberman VA, Weiss SR, Bröl J, Minne HW, Quan H, Bell NH, Rodriguez-Portales J, Downs RW, Dequeker J, Favus M. Effect of oral

alendronate on bone mineral density and the incidence of fractures in post-menopausal osteoporosis. N Engl J Med 1995; 333:1437–1443.

52. Black DM, Cummings SR, Karpf DB, Cauley JA, Thompson DE, Nevitt MC, Bauer DC, Genant HK, Haskell WL, Marcus R, Ott SM, Torner JC, Quandt SA, Reiss TF, Ensrud KE. Randomized trial of effect of alendronate on risk of fracture in women with existing vertebral fractures. Lancet 1996; 348:1535–1541.

53. Cummings SR, Black DM, Thompson DE, Applegate WB, Barrett-Connor E, Musliner TA, Palermo L, Prineas R, Rubin SM, Scott JC, Vogt T, Wallace R, Yates AJ, LaCroix AZ. Effect of alendronate on risk of fractures in women with low bone density but without vertebral fractures: results from the fracture interration trial. JAMA 1998; 280: 2077–2082.

54. Schnitzer T, Bone HG, Crepaldi G, Adami S, McClung M, Kiel D, Felsenberg D, Recker RR, Tonino RP, Roux C, Pinchera A, Foldes AJ, Greenspan SL, Levine MA, Emkey R, Santora AC II, Kaur A, Thompson DE, Yates J, Orloff JJ. Therapeutic equivalence of alendronate 70 mg once-weekly and alendronate 10 mg daily in the treatment of osteoporosis. Aging (Milano) 2000; 12:1–12.

55. Harris ST Watts NB. Genant HK, McKeever CD, Hangartner T, Keller M, Chesnut CH III, Brown J, Eriksen EF, Hoseyni MS, Axelrod DW, Miller PD. Effects of risedronate treatment on vertebral and non vertebral fractures in women with post-menopausal osteoporosis: a randomized controlled trial. Vertebral efficacy with risedronate therapy (VERT) study group. JAMA 1999; 282:1344–1352.

56. McClung MR, Geusens P, Miller PD, Zippel H, Bensen WG, Roux C, Adami S, Fogelman I, Diamond T, Eastell R, Meunier PJ, Reginster J-Y. for the Hip Intervention Program Study Group. Effect of risedronate on the risk of hip fracture in elderly women. N Engl J Med 2001; 344: 333–340.

57. Chesnut CH III, Silverman S, Andriano K, Genant H, Gimona A, Harris S, Kiel D, LeBoff M, Maricic M, Miller P, Moniz C, Peacock M, Richardson P, Watts N, Baylink D. A randomized trial of nasal spray salmon calcitonin in postmenopausal women with established osteoporosis: the prevent recurrence of osteoporotic fractures. PROOF Study Group. Am J Med 2000; 109:267–276.

58. Pun KK, Chan CWL. Analgesic effect of intranasal salmon calcitonin in the treatment of osteoporotic vertebral fractures. Clin Ther 1989; 11: 205–209.

59. Wimalawansa SJ. A four year randomized controlled trial of hormone

replacement and bisphosphonate, alone or in combination, in women with post-menopausal osteoporosis. Am J Med 1998; 104: 219–226.

60. Lindsay R, Cosman F, Lobo RA, Cosman F, Lobo RA, Walsh BW, Harris ST, Reagan JE, Liss CL, Melton ME, Byrnes CA. Addition of alendronate to ongoing hormone replacement therapy in the treatment of osteoporosis: a randomized, controlled clinical trial. J Clin Endocrinol Metab 1999; 84:3076–3081.

61. Mamelle M, Meunier PJ, Dusan R, Guillaume M, Martin JL, Gaucher A, Prost A, Zeigler G, Netter P. Risk benefit ratio of sodium fluoride treatment in primary vertebral osteoporosis. Lancet 1988; ii:361–365.

62. Riggs BL, Hodgson SF, O'Fallon WM, Chao EY, Wahner HW, Muhs JM, Cedel SL, Melton LJ III. Effect of fluoride treatment on the fracture rate in post menopausal osteoporosis. N Engl J Med 1990; 322:802–809.

63. Barnard R, Ng KW, Martin TJ, Waters MJ. Growth hormone (GH) receptor in clonal osteoblast-like cells mediate a mitogenic response to GH. Endocrinology 1991; 128:1459–1404.

64. Harris WH, Heany RP. Effect of growth hormone on skeletal mass in adult dogs. Nature 1969; 273:403–404.

65. Holloway L, Kohlmeier L, Kent K, Marcus R. Skeletal effects of cyclic recombinant human growth hormone and salmon calcitonin in osteopenic post-menopausal women. J Clin Endocrinol Metab 1997; 82:1111–1117.

66. Brown EM. Homeostatic mechanisms regulating extracellular and intracellular calcium metabolism. In: Bilezikian, Marcus, Levine, eds. The Parathyroids. New York: Raven Press, 1999: Chapter 2.

67. Tam CS, Heersche JN, Murray TM, Parsons JA. Parathyroid hormone stimulates the bone apposition rate independently of its resorptive action: differential effect of intermittent and continuous administration. Endocrinology 1982; 110:506–512.

68. Finkelstein TS. Pharmacologic mechanisms of therapeutics: Parathyroid hormone. In: Bilezekian JP, Raisz LG, Rodan GA, eds. Principles of Bone Biology. New York: Academic Press, 1996: Chapter 71.

69. Gunness-Hey M, Hock JM. Increased trabecular bone mass in rats treated with human synthetic parathyroid hormone. Metab Bone Dis Relat Res 1984; 5:177–181.

70. Moselkilde L, Sogaard CH, Danielsen CC, Torring O. The anabolic effects of human parathyroid hormone (hPTH) on rat vertebral body mass are also reflected on the quality of bone, assessed by biomechanical test-

ing: a comparison study between hPTH [1–34] and hPTH [1–84]. Endocrinology 1991; 129: 421–428.

71. Bradbeer JN, Alart ME, Meunier PJ, Reeve J. Treatment of osteoporosis with parathyroid peptide (hPTH 1–34) and estrogen: increase in volumetric density of ilia cancellous bone may depend on reduced trabecular spacing as well as increased thickness of packets of newly formed bone. Clin Endocrinol 1992; 37:282–289.

72. Neer R, Daly M, Lo C, Potts J, Nussbaum S. Treatment of postmenopausal osteoporosis with daily parathyroid hormone plus calcitriol. Third International Symposium on Osteoporosis 1990; 3:1314–1317.

73. Slovik DM, Rosenthal DI, Doppelt Sh, Potts JT, Daly MA, Campbell JA, Neer RM. Restoration of spinal bone in osteoporotic men by treatment with human parathyroid hormone [1–34] and 1,25 dihydroxyvitamin D. J Bone Miner Res 1986; 1:377–381.

74. Finkelstein JS, Klibanski A, Schaefer EH, Hornstein MD, Schiff I, Neer RM. Parathyroid hormone for the prevention of bone loss induced by estrogen deficiency. N Engl J Med 1994; 331:1618–1623.

75. Hodsman AB, Fraher LJ, Watson PH, Ostbye T, Stitt LW, Adachi JD, Taves DH, Drost D. A randomized controlled trial to compare the efficacy of cyclical parathyroid hormone versus cyclical parathyroid hormone and sequential calcitonin to improve bone mass in postmenopausal women with osteoporosis. J Clin Endocrinol Metab 1997; 82:620–628.

76. Lindsay R, Nieves J, Formica C, Henneman E, Woelfert L, Shen V, Dempster D, Cosman F. Randomized controlled study of effect of parathyroid hormone on vertebral–bone mass and fracture incidence among postmenopausal women on estrogen with osteoporosis. Lancet 1997; 350:550–555.

77. Neer RM, Arnaud CD, Zanchetta JR, Prince R, Gaich GA, Reginster A, Hodsman AB, Eriksen EF, Ish-Shalom S, Genant HK, Wang O, Mitlak BH. Effect of recombinant parathyroid hormone [1–34] on fractures and bone mineral density in post-menopausal women with osteoporosis. N Engl J Med 2001; 344:1434–1441.

78. Jaglal SB, Kreiger N, Darlington G. Past and recent physical activity and risk of hip fracture. Am J Epidemiol 1993; 138:107–118.

79. Nelson ME, Fiatarone MA, Morganti CM, Trice I, Greenberg RA, Evans WJ. Effects of high intensity strength training on multiple risk factors for osteoporotic fractures. A randomized controlled trial. JAMA 1994; 272:1909–1914.

6

In Vitro Maturation of Oocytes for Infertility Treatment

Timothy J. Child
John Radcliffe Hospital, Oxford, England

Seang Lin Tan
McGill University and McGill University Health Centre, Montreal, Quebec, Canada

I. INTRODUCTION

Since the birth of Louise Brown in 1978, the first child conceived as a result of in vitro fertilization (IVF) [1], the focus in assisted conception has been on the maturation of oocytes in vivo followed by their in vitro fertilization. It is often not recognized that prior to the early 1970s, research focused instead on the maturation in vitro of immature oocytes. As long ago as 1935, Pincus reported the spontaneous maturation under in vitro culture conditions of immature oocytes [2]. These observations were confirmed and extended by Edwards during the 1960s culminating in the maturation and fertilization in vitro of human oocytes [3,4].

The difficulties involved with the harvesting of immature oocytes, which required an ovarian biopsy through a laparotomy incision, and the low fertilization rate of in vitro matured oocytes, led to the move toward laparoscopic needle aspiration of mature oocytes from ripe ovarian follicles during stimulated menstrual cycles [5].

Although research continued during the 1970s and 1980s, it was not until 1991 that the first human pregnancy from an in vitro matured oocyte was reported [6]. This oocyte was taken from an ovary at the time of cesarean section, matured in vitro, donated to another woman, and fertilized by her partner's sperm in vitro. However, it was Trounson and colleagues who placed IVM firmly in the clinical realm when they developed an outpatient technique for immature oocyte retrieval using a specially designed aspiration needle manipulated under transvaginal ultrasound guidance [7]. During the early and mid-1990s the maturation, fertilization, and implantation rates of immature oocytes were disappointingly low, with very few reported pregnancies. It has only been in the last few years that the clinical and laboratory requirements for successful in vitro maturation (IVM) have been refined to an extent that IVM can be offered as a viable treatment alternative to stimulated IVF. Some centers are now reporting pregnancy rates per cycle for women with polycystic ovaries of 25–30% [8–10].

The aim of this review chapter is to explain the clinical and laboratory management of unstimulated IVM treatment cycles. The scientific basis of IVM will be discussed, as will the advantages of IVM treatment over stimulated IVF. Each of the steps of an IVM cycle from the immature oocyte retrieval to the embryo transfer procedure will be examined, and the rationale for each procedure given.

II. OOCYTE MATURATION

Human oocytes usually become arrested in prophase I of meiosis during fetal life [11]. At birth, the oocytes remain in the dictyate phase and each ovary has around 500,000 healthy nongrowing or primordial follicles. Throughout the reproductive life of the woman, cohorts of oocytes are removed from this nongrowing pool and commence growth. Near the completion of growth, oocytes acquire the ability to reinitiate meiosis. Following resumption of meiosis, the nuclear membrane dissolves (germinal vesicle breakdown) and chromosomes progress from metaphase I to telophase I. The completion of the first meiotic division is characterized by the extrusion of the first polar body and formation of the secondary oocyte, both of which contain a haploid chromosome complement. The second meiotic division is initiated rapidly after completion of the first and the oocytes reach metaphase II prior to ovulation. Oocyte maturation is defined as the reinitiation and completion of the first meiotic division from the germinal vesicle stage to metaphase II, with accompanying cytoplasmic maturation necessary for fertilization and early embryonic development [11].

III. ADVANTAGES OF OOCYTE IN VITRO MATURATION OVER OVARIAN STIMULATION FOR IN VITRO FERTILIZATION

To achieve high pregnancy rates with IVF treatment, gonadotropin ovarian stimulation is used to increase the number of mature oocytes retrieved, and therefore, embryos available for transfer. However, there are a number of disadvantages of gonadotropin stimulation, including high drug costs, the inconvenience of daily injections, and symptoms

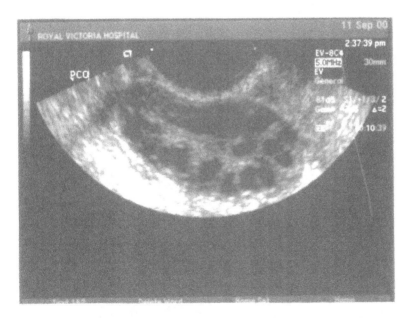

Figure 1   Early follicular phase transvaginal ultrasound scan photograph of a polycystic ovary. Note the numerous small cysts placed circumferentially around a thickened echo dense stroma.

Table 1 Results of 107 Age and Diagnosis Matched IVM and IVF Treatment Cycles for Infertile Women with PCO

	IVM	IVF	OR (95% CI)
N cycles	107	107	
Age	32.8 ± 4.2	33.1 ± 4.1	
Total injected gonadotropin units (ampules)	0	2355 ± 833 (31.4 ± 11.1)*	
Oocytes collected	10.3 ± 7.6	14.9 ± 6.5*	
Metaphase II stage oocytes	7.8 ± 4.9	12.0 ± 5.4*	
Fertilized 2PN embryos	6.1 ± 3.8	9.3 ± 4.4*	
Cleaving 2PN embryos	5.8 ± 3.7	8.6 ± 4.2*	
Embryos transferred (range)	3.2 ± 0.9 (1–5)	2.7 ± 0.8 (1–6)*	
Pregnant [N(%)]	28 (26.2%)	41 (38.3%)	0.57 (0.31–1.06)
Implantation rate [%]	9.5%	17.1%*	0.51 (0.31–0.84)
Live birth [N(%)]	17 (15.9%)	28 (26.2%)	0.53 (0.26–1.10)
Multiple live birth [N (% of total LB)]	7 (41.2%)	10 (37.0%)	1.26 (0.30–5.11)
Twins [N]	6	9	
Triplets [N]	1	1	
Moderate/severe OHSS	0	12 (11.2%)*	

Results are mean ± SD. unless stated.
* p < 0.01.

such as bloating, breast tenderness, nausea, and potentially most seriously, ovarian hyperstimulation syndrome (OHSS) [12,13]. In addition, concerns exist about a possible link between ovarian stimulation and an increased long-term risk of ovarian cancer [14]. The retrieval of oocytes from unstimulated ovaries is therefore an attractive treatment option.

We performed a case-controlled study to evaluate the viability of IVM as a treatment for women with ovaries of polycystic morphology who required assisted conception (unpublished data). An ovary was defined as polycystic (PCO) when on early follicular phase transvaginal ultrasound scan, more than 10 small (2–8 mm) follicles were present arranged around or scattered through an enlarged echodense stroma (Fig. 1). One hundred seven IVM cycles performed in 83 women with PCO were matched with 107 IVF cycles in 81 women of the same age and infertility diagnosis. The main outcomes are shown in Table 1. On average, an unstimulated IVM cycle resulted in 7.8 metaphase II oocytes and 6.1 embryos per retrieval, as compared to 12.0 metaphase II oocytes and 9.3 embryos in the IVF group ($P < 0.01$). The IVM pregnancy and live birth rates were 26.2% and 15.9% compared to 38.3% and 26.2%, respectively, for IVF (not significant). The implantation rate of IVF-derived embryos was higher (17.1% vs. 9.5% for IVM embryos [$P < 0.01$]). There were 12 (11.2%) cases of moderate to severe OHSS in the IVF group compared to none in the IVM group ($P < 0.01$). Because at least 30% of infertility patients have PCO on ultrasound [15], our results suggest that IVM is a useful treatment option.

IV. THE STAGES OF OOCYTE IN VITRO MATURATION TREATMENT

A. Overview of an IVM Treatment Cycle

The following discussion details the management of IVM as performed in our center [9]. The rationale for each procedure will then be examined.

Women with amenorrhea receive vaginal progesterone (Prometrium) 300 mg once daily for 10 days in order to induce a withdrawal bleed. All women undergo a baseline ultrasound scan on day 2–4 of menstrual bleeding to ensure that no ovarian cysts are present. Transvaginal ultrasound scans are repeated on the day of human chorionic gonadotropin (HCG) administration (see below) to exclude the development of a dominant follicle. All follicles have to be <10 mm diameter in order to proceed to oocyte retrieval, which is performed between day 9 and 14 of the cycle. Patients receive 10,000 IU HCG (Profasi) subcutaneously 36 hr before oocyte retrieval. Human chorionic gonadotropin priming increases both the percentage and rate of immature oocyte maturation [9].

Transvaginal ultrasound-guided oocyte collection is performed using a specially designed 17-G single-lumen aspiration needle. Aspiration of all small follicles is performed using intravenous fentanyl and midazolam with a paracervical block of 10 ml of 1% lidocaine. Follicular flushing is not performed.

Oocytes are collected in culture tubes containing warm 0.9% saline with 2 IU/ml heparin. The immature oocytes are incubated in culture dishes containing 1 ml of maturation medium, TC-199 medium supplemented with 20% heat-denatured maternal serum (56°C for 30 min), 0.25 mmol/l pyruvic acid (Sigma Chemical Co.), penicillin 50 mg/ml, streptomycin 75 mg/ml, 75 mIU/ml each of follicle-stimulating hormone (FSH) and luteinizing hormone (LH) (one ampule of the menotropin Humegon; Organon, Scarborough, Ontario, Canada) at 37°C in an atmosphere of 5% CO_2 and 95% air with high humidity. Following culture, the maturity of the oocytes is determined under the microscope at 24 and 48 hr.

Oocytes that are mature when checked are denuded of cumulus cells using finely drawn glass pipettes following 1 min of exposure to 0.1% hyaluronidase solution, and are then ready for intracytoplasmic sperm injection (ICSI). Spermatozoa for ICSI are prepared by Puresperm (Nidacon, Goteborg, Sweden) separation (95/70/50% gradients) at 400g for 20 min. Following Puresperm separation, the sperm pellet is washed twice (200g) with 2 ml of Vitrolife IVF medium (Vitrolife, Goteborg, Sweden). A single spermatozoon is injected into each metaphase II oocyte. Following ICSI, each oocyte is transferred into a 20 µl droplet of G 1.2 medium (Vitrolife). Fertilization is assessed 18 hr after ICSI for the appearance of two distinct pronuclei and two polar bodies.

Embryos are transferred on day 2 or 3 after ICSI. Because the oocytes are not matured and inseminated at the same time following maturation in culture, the developmental stages of embryos at the time of embryo transfer are often variable. Before transfer, all embryos for each patient are pooled and selected for transfer based on standard embryological criteria such as cleavage stage and morphological quality [16].

For endometrial preparation, patients receive estradiol valerate (Estrace) starting on the day of oocyte retrieval, depending on the endometrial thickness on that day. If the endometrial thickness is <6 mm, a 10-mg dose is given, and if it is >6 mm, a 6-mg dose is administered. If the endometrial thickness is <7 mm on the day of embryo transfer, it is recommended that the patient choose cryopreservation of all embryos for replacement in a later cycle. Luteal support is provided by 200 mg intravaginal progesterone (Prometrium) three times daily starting on the day of ICSI and continued, along with estradiol, until 12 weeks of gestation.

Each step of the IVM treatment cycle will now be addressed in turn, and important points discussed.

B. Immature Oocyte Retrieval and the Number of Oocytes Collected

We have found that the pregnancy rate in IVM is related to the number of immature oocytes collected (Fig. 2). This is because the number of embryos produced and available for transfer is dependent on the numbers of oocytes matured in vitro and fertilized. The transfer of multiple good-quality embryos increases the chance of pregnancy (see Embryo Transfer Section G below). An important goal in IVM is therefore to maximize the number of immature oocytes collected per retrieval procedure.

The work of Trounson and colleagues led to the development of the immature oocyte collection technique generally used today [7]. Immature oocytes are collected transvaginally under ultrasound guidance from small 2- to 8-mm diameter ovarian antral follicles using a specially designed short, single-channel needle with a short bevel. In addition, the aspiration pressure of the collecting system is reduced to 7.5

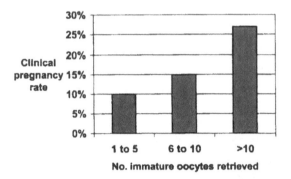

Figure 2 Graph of clinical pregnancy rate against number of immature oocytes collected in 189 consecutive unstimulated IVM treatment cycles in women with normal and polycystic ovaries ($P = 0.023$).

kPA, which is about half that used for an IVF oocyte recovery. We initially used spinal anesthesia, but have since found that good pain relief may be achieved using midazolam and fentanyl intravenous sedation in combination with a lidocaine paracervical block.

Because the pregnancy rate in IVM is related to the number of immature oocytes retrieved, it would be clinically useful to be able to predict the number of oocytes collected prior to commencing treatment. This would allow both for improved patient selection and individual counseling as to the success rate of IVM treatment. In stimulated IVF treatment a number of studies have demonstrated that a transvaginal ultrasound scan performed prior to commencing gonadotropin stimulation is able to predict the ovarian response and the number of mature oocytes retrieved. Predictive parameters include the ovarian volume [17], the total number of 2- to 8-mm antral follicles present (antral follicle count [AFC]) [18], and the maximum velocity of blood flowing through the ovarian stroma measured using transvaginal color and pulsed Doppler ultrasound [19,20].

We attempted to predict, in a prospective study, the number of immature oocytes retrieved from unstimulated ovaries during 96 unstimulated IVM treatment cycles [21]. Each woman had a transvaginal ultrasound scan performed between day 2 and 4 of the treatment cycle.

At each examination, the ovarian volume was measured and an antral follicle count performed. Finally, the maximum velocity of stromal blood flow was measured using Doppler ultrasound [19]. We found on univariate analysis that each of these three parameters was significantly predictive of the number of immature oocytes retrieved. However, after controlling for the other model factors, only the antral follicle count remained predictive of the number of immature oocytes retrieved ($P <$ 0.001). We retrieved immature oocytes from 46% of the antral follicles present at the baseline scan. An antral follicle count performed at the baseline ultrasound scan, prior to treatment, is therefore likely to be a useful predictor of outcome in IVM.

Women with ovaries of polycystic morphology by definition have more antral follicles than do women with normal ovaries. Consequently, the numbers of oocytes retrieved and the pregnancy rate in women with PCO is higher than that of women with normal ovaries [21]. IVM is therefore generally reserved for women with PCO. It does not matter whether the patient has ovulatory PCO or anovulatory polycysitic ovary syndrome (PCOS). In a comparative study, the numbers of immature oocytes collected and matured and the implantation rates were similar between women with ovulatory PCO or anovulatory PCOS (unpublished data).

It would appear logical that increasing the number of ovarian antral follicles by using mild ovarian stimulation would increase the number of retrieved immature oocytes. However, the role of ovarian stimulation in IVM is conflicting. In a randomized trial a short (3 day) or long (>3 days) protocol of recombinant FSH (rFSH) 150 mIU/day, compared with no stimulation, the number of oocytes retrieved per aspiration, or the maturation or cleavage rate did not increase [22]. This confirms the results of a previous study [23]. However, Wynn and colleagues [24] found that mild ovarian stimulation not only increased the numbers of oocytes retrieved, but also the maturation rate, though they did not perform fertilization of these oocytes. Suikkari [25] reported the luteal phase start of low-dose (37.5 mIU/day) rFSH, an approach that requires further investigation.

Some data suggest that there is a reduced retrieval rate, and therefore fewer oocytes retrieved, if a dominant follicle of >13 mm [23] or >10 mm [26] is present at the time of immature oocyte collection. Consequently, the timing of the day of oocyte recovery with regard to the presence or absence of a dominant follicle appears to be important.

C.   Timing of Immature Oocyte Retrieval

Immature oocytes may be retrieved from antral follicles and matured in vitro at all stages of the menstrual cycle, and in fact, the first IVM pregnancy resulted from immature oocytes retrieved from ovaries at the time of cesarean section [6]. However, in order to replace fresh embryos during the same cycle, and to synchronize this as closely as possible to natural conception, it is necessary to retrieve immature oocytes during the late follicular phase. In addition, as discussed above, the presence of a dominant follicle at the time of oocyte retrieval may reduce the retrieval rate. We cancel the cycle if the patient has a follicle exceeding 10 mm in diameter on the day of HCG administration, which is 2 days prior to oocyte retrieval. In a randomized, controlled trial, Cobo demonstrated that the rate of embryo development to blastocyst was significantly reduced when a dominant follicle of greater than 10 mm was present on the day of oocyte retrieval [26]. The rates of maturation and fertilization were not affected. However, others have not confirmed that the presence of a dominant follicle at the time of oocyte collection negatively affects outcome [22,27].

Recently, a Danish group examined the predictive value of the changes in estradiol and inhibin A between baseline and the day of oocyte retrieval [27]. They found no pregnancies in women with less than a doubling in estradiol concentration compared with a 19% ($P <$ 0.02) pregnancy rate in those with an estradiol increase of >100% between baseline and oocyte retrieval. When both estradiol (>100%) and inhibin A (>80%) increased in concentration, the pregnancy rate per retrieval was 24%. They suggest that measurement of these hormones may be used to help select the optimum day of immature oocyte retrieval.

D.   In Vitro Maturation

As discussed in the Introduction, it has been recognized for more than 65 years that immature oocytes can mature under in vitro culture conditions [2]. Experiments with both human and nonhuman oocytes have led to the development of culture media containing the nutrients and the conditions required for high rates of in vitro maturation.

It has been noted that immature oocytes retrieved from small follicles in ovaries stimulated for IVF mature in vitro more rapidly than do oocytes from unstimulated ovaries [11]. We questioned whether this could be due to the HCG priming given 36 hr before IVF oocyte collection, and whether HCG priming could increase the rate of maturation of immature oocytes retrieved as part of an unstimulated IVM cycle. We performed a trial in 17 patients with PCOS undergoing 24 IVM cycles in which women were randomized to be primed with 10,000 IU of HCG before the retrieval or not primed [9]. In no cycles were mature metaphase II oocytes retrieved. However, HCG priming significantly increased the numbers of oocytes matured at 24 hr (78.2% vs. 4.9%) and 48 hr (85.2% vs. 68.0%) of culture [9]. More recently, we have found that similarly high rates of oocyte maturation are also obtained when HCG priming is used in women undergoing IVM who have normal ovaries, or those with ovulatory PCO [28].

Both nuclear and cytoplasmic maturation, which involve a complex cascade of events, need to be closely integrated to ensure developmental competence. In IVM, nuclear maturation of oocytes may be complete, as evidenced by extrusion of the first polar body, while cytoplasmic maturation is incomplete. Maturation media containing FSH significantly increases fertilization and early embryo development [29,30] and consequently is routinely used in published IVM series. For more detailed discussion of the culture conditions required for IVM, readers are referred elsewhere [11].

E.   Fertilization of In Vitro Matured Oocytes

Extremely low fertilization rates, between 30 and 40%, are usually obtained after standard insemination of in vitro matured oocytes, suggesting that ICSI is the best option, even when the sperm parameters are not impaired [31,32]. Qualitative changes, including zona hardening, occur in the zona pellucida during oocyte maturation in vitro, and may reduce the fertilization rates using conventional IVF [33]. We therefore routinely use ICSI for fertilization of IVM oocytes and obtain normal (two pronuclei) fertilization rates of 75%.

F.   Embryo Development in Culture

Previous data suggest that compared to in vivo matured oocytes, those matured in vitro have a reduced embryo development rate with increased blockage of cleavage at the zygote stage [34]. However, in the case-controlled study described above in which 107 IVM cycles were age- and diagnosis-matched with 107 IVF cycles for women with PCO, we found no significant difference in fertilization or cleavage rates between in vitro and in vivo matured oocytes.

G.   Embryo Transfer and Implantation

The final step of an IVM cycle is the selection of multiple embryos for transfer to the uterine cavity. At this stage of treatment, the chance of an embryo implanting depends on a combination of embryo quality, both morphological and genetic, and the receptivity of the uterus to implantation.

To examine the effect of female age on implantation rate of IVM-produced embryos, we examined the outcome of 175 embryo transfers (unpublished data). We found that with increasing female age there was a decrease in implantation rate, presumably due to increasing oocyte aneuploidy with increasing female age (Fig. 3). This mirrors the findings in both IVF and spontaneous conceptions [35].

We also the assessed the influence of embryo quality and number transferred on pregnancy rate by means of the cumulative embryo score (CES) [16]. The CES at each embryo transfer procedure was calculated as follows. On the day of transfer the embryos were scored as grade 4, equal-sized symmetrical blastomeres; grade 3, uneven blastomeres with <10% fragmentation; grade 2, 10–50% blastomeric fragmentation; and grade 1, >50% blastomeric fragmentation. The grade of each embryo was multiplied by the number of blastomeres to produce a quality score of each embryo. The scores of all embryos transferred per patient were added to obtain the CES [16]. We found a significant relationship between the CES and the pregnancy rate ($P < 0.001$) (Fig. 4). This relationship persisted after adjusting for the numbers of embryos

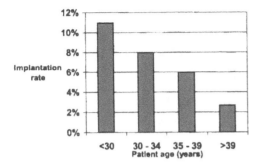

Figure 3   Graph of implantation rate of IVM-produced embryos against female age in 175 unstimulated IVM cycles ($P = 0.065$). Implantation rate is calculated as the total number of gestation sacs seen on transvaginal ultrasound scan at 6 weeks gestation divided by the total number of embryos transferred in each age category.

transferred in each CES category ($P = 0.008$), demonstrating that the grade of each embryo transferred was of prime importance.

During in vivo conception in the natural menstrual cycle, the endometrium is partially primed for implantation by endogenous estrogen produced by granulosa cells within the dominant ovarian follicle. During a stimulated IVF cycle, estrogen is produced endogenously from the numerous mature follicles produced secondary to gonadotropin stimulation. However, during an IVM cycle, a mature dominant follicle

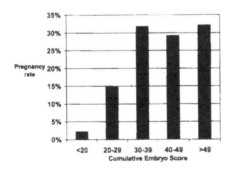

Figure 4   Graph of pregnancy rate against cumulative embryo score (CES) for 175 consecutive unstimulated IVM cycles ($P < 0.001$).

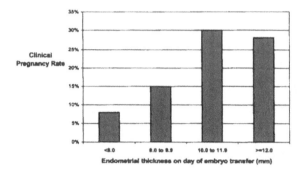

Figure 5 Graph of clinical pregnancy rate against endometrial thickness on the day of embryo transfer in 130 unstimulated IVM cycles ($P < 0.05$).

does not develop because needle aspiration is performed, and so exogenous estrogen must be administered. Russell examined the role of early or late exogenous estradiol priming of the endometrium prior to immature oocyte retrieval [36]. He found that prolonged endometrial priming prior to immature oocyte retrieval was deleterious to oocyte quality and developmental potential. We therefore commence estrogen priming from the day of oocyte retrieval in a dose dependent on endometrial thickness, and have found this approach satisfactory [9].

We have also investigated uterine receptivity to embryo implantation using transvaginal ultrasonographic measurement of the endometrial thickness. We found that the implantation rate is positively related to the endometrial thickness on the day of embryo transfer (Fig. 5).

VI. IN VITRO MATURATION FOR WOMEN WITH NORMAL OVARIES, POLYCYSTIC OVARIES, AND POLYCYSTIC OVARY SYNDROME

Because the pregnancy rate with IVM is related to the numbers of immature oocytes retrieved, and because this is most significantly related to the number of antral follicles present in the ovaries, women with polycystic ovaries are ideally suited to IVM treatment. Compared to normal ovaries, polycystic ovaries are larger, have multiple small cysts placed circumferentially around a thickened stroma (Fig. 1), and have a higher intra-ovarian stromal blood flow velocity [19]. We know that polycystic ovaries are commonly found in women presenting with infertility and that the response of women with PCO to induction of ovulation is different compared to that of women with normal ovaries [12]. The presence of PCO is an important risk factor for development of OHSS.

Many women with PCO have regular ovulatory cycles with none of the stigmata associated with PCOS, such as anovulation, hirsutism, or serum biochemical abnormalities. The large majority of published

Table 2 Results of 177 IVM Cycles in Women with Normal Ovaries (Group 1), Ovulatory PCO (Group 2), or PCOS (Group 3)

	Group 1 (normal ovaries)	Group 2 (PCO)	Group 3 (PCOS)
N patients (N cycles)	46 (56)	43 (53)	52 (68)
Age (years)	36.0 ± 3.8[a]	32.8 ± 4.1	32.9 ± 4.1
Duration of infertility (years)	5.4 ± 4.0	4.3 ± 2.9	4.5 ± 3.3
N immature oocytes	5.1 ± 3.7[a]	10.0 ± 5.1	11.3 ± 9.0
N metaphase II oocytes	4.0 ± 2.8[a]	7.6 ± 4.0	8.7 ± 5.6
N oocytes fertilized	2.9 ± 2.0[a]	5.8 ± 2.9	6.9 ± 4.5
N cleaving 2 pronuclear embryos	2.7 ± 2.0[a]	5.5 ± 2.7	6.3 ± 4.5
N embryos transferred (per transfer)	2.6 ± 1.2[a]	3.3 ± 0.9	3.2 ± 0.8
Pregnancy rate per transfer	4.0% (2 of 50)[b]	23.1% (12 of 52)	29.9% (20 of 67)
Implantation rate	1.5% (2 of 130)[b]	8.9% (15 of 169)	9.6% (21 of 220)
Livebirth rate	2% (1 of 50)[a]	17.3% (9 of 52)	14.9% (10 of 67)

Women with ovulatory PCO had ovaries of polycystic morphology on transvaginal ultrasound in the presence of regular ovulatory cycles. Women with PCOS had polycystic ovaries on ultrasound with in addition chronic anovulation and/or clinical or biochemical evidence of hirsutism.

Results are means ± SD or % (N), except as noted.

[a] $P < 0.05$ compared to groups 2 and 3.

[b] $P < 0.01$ compared to groups 2 and 3.

IVM pregnancies have been for women with PCOS. We wished to examine whether similar oocyte retrieval, maturation, fertilization, implantation, and pregnancy rates could be achieved in women with ovulatory PCO [37]. Women with normal ovaries by definition have fewer antral follicles present than do women with PCO, and would be expected to have lower numbers of oocytes retrieved. However, we also wished to assess the maturation, fertilization, implantation, and pregnancy rates in this group of women.

Our study included 177 cycles of IVM in 141 women [37]. Fifty-six of the cycles were for women with normal ovaries, 53 for women with ovulatory PCO, and 68 for women with PCOS. The main results are given in Table 2. We found no differences in any of the outcome parameters between women with ovulatory PCO and those with PCOS. In particular, the numbers of oocytes retrieved was similar. This is an important point because without a transvaginal ultrasound scan performed as part of the infertility workup, the presence of PCO in these women with regular ovulatory cycles would be missed. These women may not then have been given the option to undergo IVM treatment [37].

We have also found that, although oocytes were retrieved and embryos produced in women with normal ovaries, the implantation and pregnancy rates were low (Table 2). This finding confirmed that of previous published reports.

VI. IN VITRO MATURATION FOR OOCYTE DONATION

For a number of women, IVF is not possible using their own oocytes. This may be because of premature menopause, advanced age, or genetic or ovarian disease. The main treatment option for these women is oocyte donation. Unfortunately, there is a severe shortage of women willing to undergo the ovarian stimulation required in order to donate their oocytes to others. Because IVM is a much simpler and less invasive treatment, it may increase the pool of oocyte donors. Currently, IVM success is generally limited to women with PCO. We recently reported our experience with three women with PCO who donated their immature oocytes to other women [28]. Though there was one pregnancy, it unfortunately ended in miscarriage. In the future, IVM may increase the number of women who would consider acting as oocyte donors.

VII. IN VITRO MATURATION FOR POOR RESPONDERS TO OVARIAN STIMULATION FOR IVF

Women undergoing IVF treatment who exhibit a poor ovarian response to gonadotropin stimulation present a challenge for reproductive physicians. Such cycles typically result in a markedly reduced number of follicles, oocytes, and embryos, and consequently, a lower rate of pregnancy. Different strategies for managing subsequent treatment cycles include the gonadotropin-releasing hormone (GnRH) agonist flare protocol, microdose GnRH agonist, the use of GnRH antagonists rather than agonists, natural cycle IVF, or oocyte donation. None of these management strategies, however, is entirely satisfactory.

We hypothesized that, although the number of oocytes and embryos produced in an IVM cycle in a woman with normal ovaries and who is a poor responder to ovarian stimulation may be low, the number produced may be similar or greater than that produced in a "poor response" IVF cycle. If so, IVM could offer an alternative to an additional stimulated IVF cycle in women who are IVF poor responders.

In a preliminary study, we compared the outcome for women who had a poor response to high-dose gonadotropin stimulation for IVF in one cycle, and who, in their next cycle, underwent IVM treatment [38]. Women who had undergone IVF treatment and who had shown a poor response to ovarian stimulation with a long GnRH agonist protocol were recruited. Poor response was defined as a cycle abandoned before oocyte retrieval (≤ 4 follicles) or ≤ 4 oocytes collected at oocyte retrieval. All women had normal ovaries detected on ultrasound examination in the early follicular phase prior to commencing treatment.

The outcome variables were the number of mature oocytes and embryos produced. The CES was calculated for each transfer. Eight women with a history of poor response to IVF underwent IVM treatment. The outcomes of the treatment cycles are summarized in Table 3.

Table 3 Summary of Outcome of Eight IVM Cycles in Eight Women with a Poor Response to Ovarian Stimulation for IVF

	IVF	IVM
Number of cycles commenced	8	8
Age (years) (mean ± SD)	35.8 ± 4.0	36.8 ± 4.1
Number of cycles reaching oocyte retrieval	6	8
Number of immature oocytes	0.2 ± 0.4	1.9 ± 1.3ª
Number of mature oocytes	2.1 ± 1.6	1.8 ± 1.0
Number of embryos	1.0 ± 1.1	1.4 ± 1.2
Number of cycles reaching embryo transfer	5	6
Number of embryos transferred	1.2 ± 0.5	1.7 ± 1.0
Cumulative embryo score	11.2 ± 7.4	13.7 ± 12.4
Clinical pregnancies (%)	0	1 (12.5%)

ª $P < 0.01$.

The median (range) number of previous IVF cycles was 2.5 (1–5). The mean day 3 serum FSH concentration was 8.1 ± 2.9 IU/l. All had an FSH <12 IU/l. Six women in the IVF group reached oocyte retrieval (an additional two were cancelled before retrieval, after 9 and 17 days of stimulation, due to poor follicular response), and five women had embryos available for transfer (Table 3). During IVF stimulation, a median (range) of 5775 (3300–8400) IU of gonadotropins was used. All eight IVM cycles reached oocyte retrieval. There were similar outcomes in terms of numbers of mature oocytes, fertilized oocytes, embryos transferred, and CES between the IVF and IVM groups. There was one clinical pregnancy (gestation sac with fetal heart activity) in the IVM group that ended in miscarriage at 9 weeks gestation.

In this study, the number of embryos available, and the average cumulative embryo score following IVM were comparable to that in the previous IVF cycle. Even if IVM only produced a comparable outcome to conventional IVF in poor responders, it would have advantages as an alternative treatment because it avoids the large expense of high-dose gonadotropin therapy and its potential concomitant side effects. IVM could potentially be a useful treatment option in view of the lack of clearly superior treatment alternatives [38]. Further investigation with much larger series of patients will be required to test this hypothesis.

VIII. FUTURE DEVELOPMENTS

IVM is an exciting development in the field of assisted reproduction. However, implantation and pregnancy rates of IVM-derived embryos are relatively low compared to those produced through stimulated IVF. Consequently, numerous immature oocytes need to be retrieved, which generally restricts IVM treatment to those women with many antral follicles who have ovaries of polycystic morphology. Ongoing research should lead to improvements in the quality of in vitro matured oocytes and to an improved implantation rate. Fewer immature oocytes would then need to be retrieved, allowing women with normal ovaries to be offered this form of treatment. In addition, it is vital that the health and normality of babies born through IVM technology be carefully followed up and assessed. Worldwide, the numbers of IVM babies are still fairly few but are bound to increase greatly in the next few years.

IX. CONCLUSIONS

We have shown that the in vitro maturation of immature oocytes retrieved from unstimulated ovaries is a viable treatment alternative to stimulated IVF for women with polycystic ovaries. Advantages of IVM include reduction in cost and medical risks, particularly the risk of ovarian hyperstimulation syndrome. In addition, there is increased patient acceptability. The pregnancy rate is related to the numbers of immature oocytes retrieved that may be predicted with pretreatment transvaginal ultrasound assessment of the antral follicle count [21]. Currently, treatment is limited to those women with polycystic ovaries, who have numerous antral follicles on ultrasound. It does not matter whether the patient has additional features of PCOS such as chronic anovulation or hirsutism [37]. IVM may also increase the number of oocyte donors [28] and be a treatment option for women with a poor follicular response to ovarian stimulation for IVF [38]. In the future, improvements in the laboratory and clinical techniques of IVM should lead to increases in pregnancy rates and allow the treatment for women with normal ovaries.

REFERENCES

1. Steptoe PC, Edwards RG. Birth after the reimplantation of a human embryo. Lancet 1978; 2:366.
2. Pincus G, Enzmann EV. The comparative behaviour of mammalian eggs *in vivo* and *in vitro*. I. The activation of ovarian eggs. J Exp Med 1935; 62:655–675.
3. Edwards RG. Maturation in vitro of human ovarian oocytes. Lancet 1965; 2:926–929.
4. Edwards RG, Bavister BD, Steptoe PC. Early stages of fertilization in vitro of human oocytes matured in vitro. Nature 1969; 221:632–635.
5. Steptoe PC, Edwards RG. Laparoscopic recovery of preovulatory human oocytes after priming of ovaries with gonadotrophins. Lancet 1970; 1: 683–689.
6. Cha KY, Koo JJ, Ko JJ, Choi DH, Han SY, Yoon TK. Pregnancy after in vitro fertilization of human follicular oocytes collected from nonstimulated cycles, their culture in vitro and their transfer in a donor oocyte program. Fertil Steril 1991; 55:109–113.
7. Trounson A, Wood C, Kausche A. In vitro maturation and the fertilization and developmental competence of oocytes recovered from untreated polycystic ovarian patients. Fertil Steril 1994; 62:353–362.
8. Chian RC, Gulekli B, Buckett WM, Tan SL. Priming with human chorionic gonadotropin before retrieval of immature oocytes in women with infertility due to the polycystic ovary syndrome. N Engl J Med 1999; 341:1624, 1626.
9. Chian RC, Buckett WM, Tulandi T, Tan SL. Prospective randomized study of human chorionic gonadotrophin priming before immature oocyte retrieval from unstimulated women with polycystic ovarian syndrome. Hum Reprod 2000; 15:165–170.
10. Cha KY, Han SY, Chung HM, Choi DH, Lim JM, Lee WS, Ko JJ, Yoon TK. Pregnancies and deliveries after in vitro maturation culture followed by in vitro fertilization and embryo transfer without stimulation in women with polycystic ovary syndrome. Fertil Steril 2000; 73:978–983.

11. Cha KY, Chian RC. Maturation in vitro of immature human oocytes for clinical use. Hum Reprod Update 1998; 4:103–120.

12. MacDougall MJ, Tan SL, Balen A, Jacobs HS. A controlled study comparing patients with and without polycystic ovaries undergoing in-vitro fertilization. Hum Reprod 1993; 8:233–237.

13. Engmann L, Maconochie N, Sladkevicius P, Bekir J, Campbell S, Tan SL. The outcome of in-vitro fertilization treatment in women with sonographic evidence of polycystic ovarian morphology. Hum Reprod 1999; 14:167–171.

14. Whittemore AS. The risk of ovarian cancer after treatment for infertility. N Engl J Med 1994; 331:805–806.

15. Kousta E, White DM, Cela E, McCarthy MI, Franks S. The prevalence of polycystic ovaries in women with infertility. Hum Reprod 1999; 14: 2720–2723.

16. Steer CV, Mills CL, Tan SL, Campbell S, Edwards RG. The cumulative embryo score: a predictive embryo scoring technique to select the optimal number of embryos to transfer in an in-vitro fertilization and embryo transfer programme. Hum Reprod 1992; 7:117–119.

17. Lass A, Skull J, McVeigh E, Margara R, Winston RM. Measurement of ovarian volume by transvaginal sonography before ovulation induction with human menopausal gonadotrophin for in-vitro fertilization can predict poor response. Hum Reprod 1997; 12:294–297.

18. Ng EH, Tang OS, Ho PC. The significance of the number of antral follicles prior to stimulation in predicting ovarian responses in an IVF programme. Hum Reprod 2000; 15:1937–1942.

19. Zaidi J, Barber J, Kyei-Mensah A, Bekir J, Campbell S, Tan SL. Relationship of ovarian stromal blood flow at the baseline ultrasound scan to subsequent follicular response in an in vitro fertilization program. Obstet Gynecol 1996; 88:779–784.

20. Engmann L, Sladkevicius P, Agrawal R, Bekir J, Campbell S, Tan SL. The pattern of changes in ovarian stromal and uterine artery blood flow velocities during in vitro fertilization treatment and its relationship with outcome of the cycle. Ultrasound Obstet Gynecol 1999; 13:26–33.

21. Child TJ, Gulekli B, Tan SL. Success during in-vitro maturation (IVM) of oocyte treatment is dependent on the numbers of oocytes retrieved which are predicted by early follicular phase transvaginal ultrasound measurement of the antral follicle count and peak ovarian stromal blood flow velocity. Hum Reprod 2001; 16 (abstr book 1): O101.

22. Mikkelsen AL, Smith SD, Lindenberg S. In-vitro maturation of human oocytes from regularly menstruating women may be successful without

follicle stimulating hormone priming. Hum Reprod 1999; 14:1847–1851.

23. Trounson A, Anderiesz C, Jones GM, Kausche A, Lolatgis N, Wood C. Oocyte maturation. Hum Reprod 1998; 13(suppl 3):52–62.

24. Wynn P, Picton HM, Krapez JA, Rutherford AJ, Balen AH, Gosden RG. Pretreatment with follicle stimulating hormone promotes the numbers of human oocytes reaching metaphase II by in-vitro maturation. Hum Reprod 1998; 13:3132–3138.

25. Suikkari AM, Tulppala M, Tuuri T, Hovatta O, Barnes F. Luteal phase start of low-dose FSH priming of follicles results in an efficient recovery, maturation and fertilization of immature human oocytes. Hum Reprod 2000; 15:747–751.

26. Cobo AC, Requena A, Neuspiller F, Aragon s M, Mercader A, Navarro J, Simon C, Remohi J, Pellicer A. Maturation in vitro of human oocytes from unstimulated cycles: selection of the optimal day for ovum retrieval based on follicular size. Hum Reprod 1999; 14:1864–1868.

27. Mikkelsen AL, Smith S, Lindenberg S. Impact of oestradiol and inhibin A concentrations on pregnancy rate in in-vitro oocyte maturation. Hum Reprod 2000; 15:1685–1690.

28. Gulekli B, Child TJ, Chian RC, Tan SL. Immature oocytes from unstimulated polycystic ovaries: a new source of oocytes for donation. Reprod Technol 2001; 10:295–298.

29. Schroeder AC, Downs SM, Eppig JJ. Factors affecting the developmental capacity of mouse oocytes undergoing maturation in vitro. Ann N Y Acad Sci 1988; 541:197–204.

30. Jinno M, Sandow BA, Hodgen GD. Enhancement of the developmental potential of mouse oocytes matured in vitro by gonadotropins and ethylenediaminetetraacetic acid (EDTA). J In Vitro Fert Embryo Transf 1989; 6:36–40.

31. Nagy ZP, Cecile J, Liu J, Loccufier A, Devroey P, Van Steirteghem A. Pregnancy and birth after intracytoplasmic sperm injection of in vitro matured germinal-vesicle stage oocytes: case report. Fertil Steril 1996; 65:1047–1050.

32. Hwang JL, Lin YH, Tsai YL. In vitro maturation and fertilization of immature oocytes: a comparative study of fertilization techniques. J Assist Reprod Genet 2000; 17:39–43.

33. Choi TS, Mori M, Kohmoto K, Shoda Y. Beneficial effect of serum on the fertilizability of mouse oocytes matured in vitro. J Reprod Fertil 1987; 79:565–568.

34. Barnes FL, Kausche A, Tiglias J, Wood C, Wilton L, Trounson A. Pro-

duction of embryos from in vitro-matured primary human oocytes. Fertil Steril 1996; 65:1151–1156.

35. Tan SL, Royston P, Campbell S, Jacobs HS, Betts J, Mason B, Edwards RG. Cumulative conception and livebirth rates after in-vitro fertilisation. Lancet 1992; 339:1390–1394.

36. Russell JB. Immature oocyte retrieval combined with in-vitro oocyte maturation. Hum Reprod 1998; 13(suppl 3): 63–70.

37. Child TJ, Gulekli B, Abdul-Jalil AK, Tan SL. In-vitro maturation and fertilization of oocytes from unstimulated normal ovaries, polycystic ovaries, or polycystic ovarian syndrome. Fertil Steril 2001; 76:936–942.

38. Child TJ, Gulekli B, Chian RC, Abdul-Jalil AK, Tan SL. In-vitro maturation (IVM) of oocytes from unstimulated normal ovaries of women with a previous poor response to IVF. Fertil Steril 2000; 74(3S): S45.

7
Preimplantation Genetic Diagnosis

Asangla Ao
McGill University and McGill University Health Centre, Montreal, Quebec, Canada

I. INTRODUCTION

Genetic diseases affect about 3% of the human population at birth and contribute to serious illness and infant mortality. Half of these defects are caused by chromosomal abnormalities, and the other half includes genetic contributions to congenital abnormalities and other common diseases, including single gene defects. With the development of new molecular technologies and the use of assisted reproduction techniques, several inherited genetic diseases can now be diagnosed in polar body and cleavage stage human embryos. This procedure provides an alternative to prenatal diagnosis for couples at risk of transmitting genetic disorders to their children by selective transfer of only unaffected embryos to the uterus, and it avoids the possibility of termination later in gestation. The first successful clinical attempt to screen preimplantation embryos for genetic disease was achieved in 1990 by Handyside and colleagues [1] for X-linked diseases. Since then, the number of centers as well as range of diseases for genetic diagnosis have increased considerably. This has been made possible by the development of sensitive technologies to identify accurate chromosome numbers and detect genetic mutations in single cells from early embryos.

II. APPROACHES TO PREIMPLANTATION GENETIC DIAGNOSIS

Genetic analysis for preimplantation genetic diagnosis (PGD) can be performed on three cell types: polar bodies (PBs) removed from oocyte and zygote, blastomeres from a cleavage stage embryo, and on a few trophectoderm cells from a blastocyst.

Preconception genetic analysis, or the removal of and diagnosis from the first polar body, was first developed by Verlinsky and colleagues [2]. Despite some advantages, preconception genetic analysis cannot be used for paternally transmitted diseases and it is less efficient for telomeric genes. To ensure correct diagnosis, the second polar body (after fertilization) is usually removed for further analysis [3].

The most common method used for preimplantation genetic diagnosis is the biopsy and genetic analysis of cleavage stage embryos [4]. At early cleavage stages, each cell of the mammalian embryo remains totipotent and can contribute to all the tissues of the conceptus. However, each cleavage division subdivides the cytoplasm of the zygote into successively smaller cells and there appears to be a lower limit of embryo mass compatible with implantation and development. Therefore, embryo biopsy is performed as late as possible before transfers are normally carried out, early on day 3 post insemination at the 6- to 10-cell stage. Embryos are placed in drops of N-2-hydroxyethylpiperazine-N-2-ethanesulfonic acid (HEPES) buffered medium under oil and transferred to a microscope for micromanipulation. The embryo is immobilized on a flame-polished holding pipette and a hole is drilled in the zona pellucida with a stream of Tyrode acid from a fine micropipette or by using laser. A second larger micropipette is then pushed through the hole in the zona to aspirate one or two cells (Fig. 1). The biopsied embryo is then returned to culture and the biopsied cell prepared for genetic analysis.

Cleavage stage biopsy and removal of one or two cells does not adversely affect preimplantation development as assessed by the proportion of embryos developing to the blastocyst stage in vitro [5]. Also, embryo metabolism is only reduced proportional to the cell numbers, indicating that the viability of the embryos and their cleavage rates are

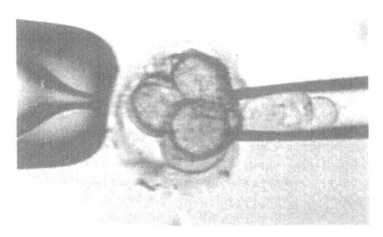

Figure 1   Human cleavage stage biopsy for preimplantation genetic diagnosis.

not affected. Removal of cells at totipotent stages should not effect postimplantation development and fetal abnormalities have not been reported following the transfer of cryopreserved embryos, in which some cells were destroyed on thawing. Approximately 200 babies have been born after cleavage stage biopsy and no increased congenital abnormalities have been reported.

Blastocyst biopsy is another method that can be used for PGD. The total number of cells increases to more than 100 at the blastocyst stage. The removal of trophectoderm cells for genetic diagnosis has the advantage over polar body and cleavage stage biopsies due to the availability of a larger number of cells without affecting the inner cell mass (ICM), which gives rise to fetus later in development. The technical challenges faced in single cell diagnosis can also be overcome by using 10–15 trophectoderm cells by this approach. Technical feasibility of blastocyst biopsy on nonclinical setup has been successful [6–9], however, so far this procedure has not been applied clinically. The low blastocyst rate in in vitro culture has been the limiting factor for this approach to be clinically viable. However, recent success in obtaining increased blastocyst rate with improved culture media and higher pregnancy rates after blastocyst transfer indicate that this approach may be suitable for selected patients [10,11].

III. GENETIC ANALYSIS ON BIOPSIED CELLS

The approach used for genetic analysis of a single cell depends upon the type of disease being investigated. For chromosomal abnormalities such as translocations, age-related aneuploidy, and sex selection, fluorescence in situ hybridization (FISH) is used. However, for single gene defects, polymerase chain reaction (PCR) is the only technique currently being used.

IV. SEX SELECTION

The demand for sex selection in embryos to avoid X-linked disease is one of the growing requests for PGD. There are reportedly 400 X-linked diseases [12] and for most of them there is no specific molecular diagnosis. The current alternatives for these patients, until more specific tests are developed, are either preimplantation diagnosis and transfer of only female embryos to the uterus, or termination of all male fetuses after prenatal diagnosis, of which half would be unaffected.

Sex selection for X-linked disorders was first employed for PGD using PCR amplification of Y-linked sequences [1]. Single blastomeres biopsied at the cleavage stage on day 3 were analyzed for the presence or absence of the Y-linked amplified fragment, and an embryo was identified as female if the expected DNA fragment was absent. However, presumably the failure of amplification of a male embryo led to misdiagnosis in one singleton pregnancy, which was subsequently terminated [13]. Co-amplification of both X- and Y-sequences was later used to overcome such problems [14], but amplification of both sequences may fail independently and cause misdiagnosis. Current use of the same primers to amplify homologous genes on the X- and Y-chromosomes, e.g., ZFX and ZFY [15], steroid sulfatase gene [16], and amelogenin gene [17], may help to avoid the failure of specific primers.

The development of interphase FISH in single cells has provided an alternative to use of PCR and is now the preferred method for sexing embryos. This approach is virtually contamination free, which is a major concern in PCR assays. In addition, unlike PCR, analysis of embryos by FISH allows the detection of copy number for each chromosome tested, thus avoiding the transfer of embryos with sex chromosome abnormalities such as Turner's syndrome (45 XO).

V. CHROMOSOME ABNORMALITY

The fecundity rate in humans is much lower than other mammals and is estimated to be 25% [18]. This low rate is explained by the high frequency of reproductive wastage before or at the time of implantation. Among the pregnancies that are recognized clinically, about 15–20% of concepti are lost as spontaneous abortions between the 6th to 28th weeks of gestation [19,20]. Extensive cytogenetic studies in this group of failed pregnancies show a chromosome abnormality rate of 50% [21], which is in contrast to only 5% of stillborns that show such chromosome abnormalities. This suggests that most of the chromosomally abnormal conceptions are lost prior to establishing a clinical pregnancy. Of the different classes of chromosome abnormalities observed in spontaneous abortions, only 2.4% are due to parental chromosome rearrangements [22]. Aneuplody (mainly trisomy) is reported to be the most common cause of pregnancy loss [23] and it is also the leading cause of mental retardation among those pregnancies that survive to term.

Chromosome abnormalities may arise during gametogenesis, fertilization, and embryogenesis. Most aneuploidies, however, arise from maternal nondisjunction and their number increases with advanced maternal age. In recent years, a growing number of research articles have been published on chromosome status in gametes and embryos due to widespread use of in vitro fertilization treatment for infertility and donated supernumerary embryos made available for research.

Most of the initial data available on oocytes and embryos were by karyotype analysis [24–32]. However, because of the difficulty in obtaining good metaphase spreads from cleaving embryos and artificial loss of chromosomes during preparation, the information obtained was limited. The present use of interphase FISH with multiple chromosome-specific DNA probes, labeled with different fluorochromes, provides an efficient and rapid analysis of numerical chromosomal imbalances in most of the cells from a cleavage stage embryo. Studies show that the rate of chromosomal errors in the early stages of embryo development is much higher than in clinically established pregnancies [33–36]. Among the chromosome anomalies observed in preimplantation embryos, a large proportion of them are chromosomally mosaic comprising cells with both diploid and nondiploid chromosome compliments [34,37–42]. Mosaicism in these embryos is of various types involving one or more chromosomes. The more diverse types of mosaicism observed in preimplantation human embryos compared to those observed in spontaneous abortions or during prenatal diagnosis may suggest that some of them are incompatible with implantation. Chromosomal mosaicism is not restricted to embryos obtained from infertile patients. A high frequency of chromosomal mosaicism has been observed in fertile patients undergoing preimplantation genetic diagnosis for X-linked disease [41]. The high rate of chromosomal abnormality observed in early human embryos led to the suggestion that an artifact of FISH analysis may have contributed to this high frequency. However, recent reports using primed in situ labeling (PRINS) [43] and karyotyping [40] gave similar results, suggesting that the high degree of mosaicism may be a natural phenomenon observed in early human embryos, although the effect of in vitro culture conditions and hormone stimulation protocol cannot be ruled out.

VI. FISH AND PGD

The ideal method for preimplantation diagnosis of chromosome abnormality in cleavage stage embryos would be karyotyping of the metaphase nucleus. However, it is not always possible to obtain good metaphase spread from cleavage stage blastomeres, and it is technically demanding; therefore, FISH is being routinely used for detecting chromosomal abnormalities in blastomeres.

Currently, in addition to sexing embryos for sex-linked diseases, FISH is also employed for preimplantation diagnosis of aneuploidy screening for women of advanced maternal age and for translocation carriers.

A.   Aneuploidy Screening

The association between increasing maternal age and higher aneuploidy rate is observed in oocytes and embryos following in vitro fertilization [35,44,45]. Fertility declines with advancing maternal age [46] and this is more apparent in women undergoing infertility treatment. Pregnancy can be achieved in older women using donated eggs from younger women, indicating that it is the aging of the egg rather than the endometrium which is responsible for the low pregnancy rate in this group of women. To improve the implantation rate in this group of patients, aneuploidy screening was introduced to select only the normal embryos for transfer. Aneuploidy screening in PBs was first applied clinically by Verlinsky and colleagues [3,47,48] using DNA probes for some of the chromosomes most commonly involved in spontaneous abortions, chromosomes X, 18, and/or 13/21. Aneuploidy screening was subsequently performed in blastomeres with an increased number of chromosome probes [49,50]. More than 100 babies have been born after aneuploidy screening in PB and blastomeres [49–53]. Recent analysis of data from aneuploidy screening in cleavage stage embryos shows an increased implantation rate among some groups of patients and an overall decrease in spontaneous abortion rate when compared with a control group [50]. However, no randomized clinical trial has been carried out on a large enough population to significantly demonstrate improved success rates with routine aneuploidy screening for women of advanced maternal age, and the debate on its benefits is still ongoing.

B.   PGD for Chromosome Translocations

Patients carrying balanced chromosomal rearrangements, although not usually infertile, may experience repeated miscarriages. This is due to the production of chromosomally unbalanced gametes. The most common structural chromosome rearrangements found in humans are robertsonian translocations. All five human acrocentric autosomes (13, 14, 15, 21, and 22) are capable of participating in robertsonian translocations and individuals carrying all 10 possible types have been reported. However, the most commonly observed translocations are between chromosomes 13 and 14, and chromosomes 14 and 21 [54]. The first successful preimplantation genetic diagnosis for two female carriers of robertsonian translocations, 45 XX, der (13;14)(q10;q10) was performed in metaphase chromosomes obtained from first polar bodies using whole chromosome painting probes [55]. In the first case, three normal embryos were transferred, resulting in normal triplets which included one set of monozygotic twins. The second patient had three embryos transferred; two normal and one chromosomally balanced and resulted in the birth of one normal and one chromosomally balanced child. Diagnoses for robertsonian translocations also have been performed in blastomeres after cleavage stage biopsy [55–57]. The most commonly found chromosome translocations in patients requesting PGD are for the carriers of balanced reciprocal translocations. Most of these reciprocal translocations are unique to the family. Similar to PGD performed for robertsonian translocations, polar body analysis can be performed for female carriers for reciprocal translocations. In the blastomere analysis, researchers have used two main approaches: designing specific probes spanning the breakpoints of the translocation or using two probes flanking the break point of the translocation [56–59]. Although PGD has been applied clinically for carriers of chromosome translocations, the number of babies born is still very small and only a few centers have been able to perform these tests, particularly because of limited numbers of commercially available probes.

VII. PGD OF SINGLE GENE DEFECTS

Progress in molecular genetic techniques has led to the identification of single gene defects responsible for inherited disorders. Thus far, more than 5000 single gene defects have been reported [60]. Carriers for single gene defects are the largest group of patients requesting preimplantation genetic diagnosis [61].

Within affected families, single gene defects are usually identified by their mendelian mode of inheritance. Although half of the single gene defects are dominant [60], many conditions show a high variability of penetrance (e.g., neurofibromatosis 1 [62]). These enable affected persons to reach reproductive age and pass on the mutation to the next generation. In contrast, autosomal-recessive disorders are only expressed when two mutations (homozygous or compound heterozygous) within the same gene have been inherited. There is a class of genetic diseases, due to single gene defects, which do not exhibit the typical pattern of mendelian inheritance. By examining affected pedigrees, it is observed that the severity of the disorder increases with each successive generation [63–65]. Recently, cloning of several of these genes has demonstrated the unique mechanism that explains their unusual inheritance. Each of these disorders has been shown to be associated with an unstable trinucleotide repeat element. Moreover, there is a correlation between the size of the repeat and the severity of the phenotype. Instability of the repeat during meiosis and mitosis results in an amplification of the repeat number. This correlation can be seen between the affected parent and affected offspring, and is often referred to as "anticipation" of the disease [66,67].

Though not used widely for sex selection, PCR is the only method sensitive enough to detect single gene mutations. Handyside and colleagues [68] were the first to develop PCR techniques to detect the cystic fibrosis (CF) ΔF508 mutation in single cells, leading to the first birth of a healthy child after PGD for cystic fibrosis. Since then, preimplantation genetic diagnosis has been offered for numerous autosomal-dominant and autosomal-recessive disorders (Table 1).

A. Techniques Used for Genetic Analysis

Autosomal-Recessive Disorders

Theoretically, PGD for any single gene defect can be developed, provided the mutation causing the disorder is well characterized. Specific DNA primers can be designed encompassing the mutation that amplify the segment by PCR to a level at which it can be visualized for genetic analysis. In recent years amplification of DNA from a single cell has improved considerably, however, a lower amplification rate is always

Table 1 Major Reported Clinical Application of PGD for Single-Gene Disorders with PCR

Disease	Gene/map locus/mutation	PGD method(s)	Main reference(s)
Autosomal recessive			
Cystic fibrosis (CF)	*CFTR* gene/7q31.2/75% of CF mutation is a 3 bp deletion, delF508	PCR/heteroduplex formation	Handyside et al. [68] Ao et al. [69]
Beta-thalassemia	Beta-hemoglobin gene/11p15.5/beta-zero (absence of beta chain) and beta-plus-(reduced amounts of detectable beta-globin)-thalassemia	(1) Restriction enzyme digestion and use of a linked marker (2) DGGE	Kuliev et al. [71] Kanavakis et al. [73]
Sickle cell anemia	Beta-hemoglobin gene/11p15.5/sixth codon GAG to GTG	Restriction enzyme digestion and use of a linked marker	Xu et al. [112]
21-Hydroxylase deficiency	21-Hydroxylase gene/6p21.3/most are deletion	Fluorescent PCR	Van de Velde et al. [113]
Tay-Sachs	*HEXA* gene/15q23-q24/heterogeneous (the reported PGDs were for 4 bp insertion and two frequent mutations, respectively)	(1) Heteroduplex formation (2) Nested duplex PCR	Gibbons et al. [114] Sermon et al. [99]
Spinal muscular atrophy type 1 (SMA 1)	*SMN1* gene/5q12.2-q13.3/disruption of telomeric copy of the gene	Nested PCR and restriction enzyme digestion	Dreesen et al. [74]

Autosomal dominant			
Myotonic dystrophy	DMPK gene/19q13.2-q13.3/ expanded CTG repeats	Fluorescent PCR	Sermon et al. [84] Sermon et al. [80]
Huntington's disease	Huntington gene/4p16.3/ expanded CAG repeats	F-multiplex PCR Fluorescent PCR	Dean et al. [88] Sermon et al. [81]
Marfan's syndrome	Fibrilin-1 gene/15q21.1/ variable mutations	(1) Use of a linked marker (radioactive) (2) Restriction digestion (3) Use of a linked marker (fluorescent PCR)	Harton et al. [90] Blaszczyk et al. [91] Sermon et al. [92]
Charcot-Marie-Tooth Type 1A	PMP22 gene/17p11.2/duplication of, or mutations in the gene (PGD for duplication)	Use of a linked marker (fluorescent PCR)	De Vos et al. [115]
Osteogenesis imperfecta types 1 and 4 (OI1 and OI4)	COLIA 1 and 2 genes/ 17q21.31-q22 and 7q22.1 heterogeneous (PGDs for COLIA1 1-bp deletion and COLIA2 G to A substitution mutation)	Fluorescent PCR	De Vos et al. [116]

Table 1 Continued

Disease	Gene/map locus/mutation	PGD method(s)	Main reference(s)
Li-Fraument syndrome (p53 tumor-suppressor mutation)	p53 Tumor-suppressor gene/17p13.1/heterogeneous (the PGD for 902ins C- and G524A)	Restriction enzyme digestion	Verlinsky et al. [117]
Autosomal dominant retinitis pigmentosum	Rhodopsin genes/heterogeneous/heterogeneous (reported PGD for C to A transversion in the gene on chromosome 7)	PCR-ADLP and SSM	Strom et al. [118]
X-linked			
Duchenne muscular dystrophy (DMD)	Dystrophin gene/Xp21.2/ about 2/3 cases are deletion of one or many exons	(1) Nested multiplex PCR (2) Use of linked markers with multiplex PCR (for nondeletion DMD)	Liu et al. [95] Lee et al. [119]
Fragile X syndrome	FMR-1 gene/Xq27.3/expanded CGG repeat	Fluorescent PCR	Sermon et al. [97]
Lesch-Nyhan syndrome	HPRT gene/Xq26-q27.2/ heterogeneous (PGD for G to C substitution)	Nested PCR and restriction enzyme digestion	Ray et al. [96]

ADLP = allele-dependent length polymorphism; SSM = site-specific mutagenesis; DGGE = denaturing gradient electrophoresis.

observed in blastomeres when compared to single lymphocytes. This is due to the sampling of blastomeres with degenerating or apoptotic nuclei, and also the inadvertent sampling of blastomeres with no nucleus. So far, the largest series of PGD performed for an autosomal-recessive disorder is for cystic fibrosis [61]. It is the most common autosomal-recessive disease among White population affecting about 1 in 2000 live births. The first clinical PGD for the major mutation causing CF (ΔF508 deletion) was performed by a nested PCR assay followed by heteroduplex analysis. This technique was sensitive and accurate enough to genotype normal, carrier, or affected embryos in single blastomeres. In a series of 22 PGD clinical cycles where both partners were carriers for ΔF508 deletion, 145 normally fertilized embryos were biopsied and genetic testing was performed using this method. In 18 cycles, one or two unaffected embryos were transferred and a total of five clinical pregnancies were established, and at birth all five singletons were confirmed as homozygous for the normal allele [69,70]. In addition to CF, a number of other tests for autosomal genetic disorders have been clinically applied (Table 1).

Restriction enzyme digestion followed by fragment analysis is another common method employed for genetic diagnosis. The mutant and normal alleles can be distinguished after the digestion with specific restriction enzymes and the product resolved by gel electrophoresis. This approach was used to genotype the sampled cells for PGD of thalassemia mutations [71,72]. In a different clinical series, Kanavakis and colleagues [73] analyzed the amplified product by denaturing gradient gel electrophoresis. This approach was successfully applied to 10 couples at risk of transmitting β-thalassemia major and six pregnancies were reported. Two pregnancies resulted in birth of two healthy singletons and three are ongoing pregnancies. One ectopic pregnancy was terminated. A naturally occurring restriction enzyme site may not be available in all cases. In such a situation, an artificial restriction enzyme site can be introduced by using a modified primer sequence and such approach was applied clinically for PGD for spinal muscular atrophy (SMA) [74], (Ao, Blake and Tan, unpublished).

The conventional methods of detecting the PCR product after gel electrophoresis have been ethidium bromide or silver staining. Alternatively, the product was labeled either with radioactive primers or nucleotides. The limitations of these methods are low sensitivity to detect the product, thus requiring a large number of PCR cycles, and poor accuracy in separating fragments of small size differences. Recent use of fluorescent PCR (F-PCR) technology in PGD has increased the sensitivity of the test considerably. Fluorescent-based DNA detection technology was first developed for automated sequencing [75] and then adapted for PCR fragment analysis and applied for genetic screening [76–81]. Incorporation of fluorescently labeled primers into PCR products enables a laser excitation/detection system to register the DNA fragments as excitation peaks, producing a system more sensitive than standard gel electrophoresis [82]. As a consequence of the increased sensitivity with fluorescent-PCR, a low allele drop-out (ADO, failure of amplification of one of the alleles) rate has been reported due to an ability to distinguish true ADO from preferential amplification of one allele [83]. Fluorescent-based systems are highly amenable to multiplex PCR, allowing the incorporation of one or more short tandem repeats (STRs) in a PCR assay to detect DNA contamination.

Autosomal-Dominant Disorders

One of the largest series of autosomal-dominant conditions to have been treated by PGD is myotonic dystrophy (DM) followed by Huntington's disease [61,80,81,84]. Both of these disorders belong to the group of trinucleotide repeat disorders, of which there are currently 14 that cause neurological disease when there is an expansion of the repeat [85]. The presence of high CG content of the expanded trinucleotide repeats makes the development of single-cell PCR assays particularly challenging. Myotonic dystrophy is the most common form of adult-onset muscular dystrophy and the unstable CTG repeat is located in the 3′ untranslated region of the myotonic dystrophy protein kinase gene (DMPK) [86,87]. The CTG repeat unit is highly heterogeneous in the unaffected general population, ranging from 5 to 37 repeats, whereas an adult-onset patient may have 100–1000 repeats and congenital cases have been reported to have up to 6000 repeats [86]. At present, the PCR protocols for DM are unable to amplify the expanded repeat at the single-cell level, so the diagnosis depends on the detection of the healthy allele from the affected parent [80,84]. However, potential couples for PGD must be informative, i.e., the healthy allele of the affected parent should have a different repeat size from that of the unaffected parent. This approach, therefore, cannot be used for all DM couples that intend to undergo PGD. An ideal situation would be to amplify both the normal and the affected alleles from the same sample. However, until such test can be developed at the single-cell level, the present approach is the only alternative.

Recently, we developed a heminested multiplex fluorescent PCR for DM to improve over the current protocol to monitor contamination and allelic drop-out, which could otherwise lead to misdiagnosis. The multiplex PCR assay for DM was designed to incorporate two highly heterozygous and closely linked STR markers from chromosome 19 (D19S559 and D19S219). The PCR assay, when tested on a large number of single lymphocytes from different individuals, including in human blastomeres, was highly accurate and efficient [88]. This approach was then used to perform PGD for a couple for DM (Fig. 2). Preclinical test showed that the marker D19S219 was informative for the couple and was incorporated into the test. The ensuing in vitro fertilization(IVF)-PGD cycle resulted in nine normally fertilized embryos that were biopsied and tested on day 3. From the 12 blastomeres tested, the amplification rate for DM was 91.7% (11 of 12) with ADO of 0%; amplification for the D19S219 STR was also 91.7% (11 of 12) but with ADO of 18.2% (2 of 11). None of the 10 blanks tested showed any amplification. Two embryos diagnosed to be unaffected were transferred to the patient, but she did not become pregnant. Tests on all nontransferred embryos confirmed results of the PGD.

In addition to DM, PGD has been successfully applied to other autosomal-dominant disorders and healthy babies were born [61,89] (Table 1). Depending upon the mutation that caused the disorders, variable strategies were used to identify normal and affected embryos. In some instances, different groups applied alternative strategies for the same disorder to perform PGD. The mutation for Marfan's syndrome was identified by using a linked marker in a radioactive PCR assay [90], restriction enzyme digestion followed by gel electrophoresis [91], and the use of linked marker by fluorescent-based PCR [92]. All of these approaches were efficient enough to distinguish between normal and affected embryos.

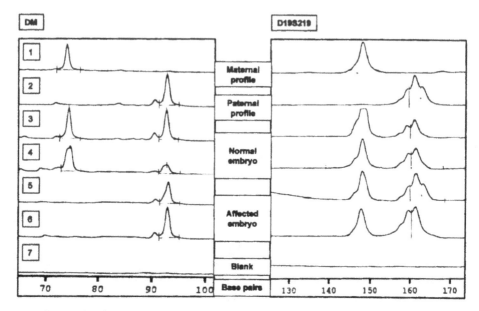

Figure 2 Representation of the results from the clinical PGD for DM and the dinucleotide STR D19S219. Results obtained after preimplantation genetic diagnosis for DM and D19S219 STR on the same blastomeres. Lane 1 shows the female profile for DM with 5 CTG repeat units and D19S219 homozygous for 10 CA repeat units. Lane 2 shows the male profile for DM with 13 CTG repeat units and D19S219 homozygous for 16 repeat units. Lanes 3 and 4 show a normal embryo. Lanes 5 and 6 show an embryo diagnosed to be affected. Lane 7 shows a blank sample.

Some diseases may manifest much later in life; for example, Huntington's disease and adenomatous polyposis coli (APC). The termination of pregnancy after conventional prenatal diagnosis for carriers of such disorders is controversial and may not be acceptable for some couples. Affected children are otherwise healthy and may remain so for many years. The first attempt at PGD for an inherited cancer predisposition syndrome was for familial adenomatous polyposis coli (FAPC), an autosomal-dominant condition characterized by the development of hundreds or thousands of colorectal adenomas and subsequent development of adenocarcinoma in all untreated cases. Despite the availability of genetic testing for APC gene mutation, there has been little interest in prenatal diagnosis among parents who are carriers for this disease. However, most parents would be keen to reduce the risk of an affected pregnancy if the option were available [93]. The PGD patient for FAPC was 34 years old and the causative mutation in the family was determined to be a T insertion at codon 764, a site that normally correlates with the classical FAPC phenotype. The biopsied cells from each of the normally fertilized embryos were first subjected to whole genome amplification by primer extension preamplification (PEP) followed by nested PCR. Two APC fragments were amplified: one included the mutation site and the other was an informative intragenic polymorphism. Both were detected by simultaneous single strand conformation polymorphism (SSCP) and heteroduplex analysis. Out of four biopsied embryos, three embryos showed APC mutation confirmed by the identification of the mutation-associated polymorphism. A single embryo diagnosed as normal for both tests was transferred to the mother, but she did not become pregnant [94]. By using two markers, the possibility of misdiagnosis, which could be serious for an autosomal-dominant condition such as APC, was greatly reduced because ADO of either allele was monitored

X-Linked Disorders

Polymerase chain reaction-based genetic diagnosis has been used for a number of X-linked diseases where the disease-causing gene is identified (Table 1). Compared to sex selection for X-linked recessive disorders, where 50% of the unaffected male embryos are discarded, specific mutation detection allows more embryos to be made available for transfer. Although initially sex selection was performed for Duchenne muscular dystrophy (DMD), the cloning of the dystrophin gene has permitted molecular analysis for PGD [95]. Similarly, sex selection for a female carrier with Lesch-Nyhan syndrome was originally attempted by sex selection. Following characterization of the family mutation, three PCR-based PGD cycles were performed. The mutation was detected by restriction enzyme digestion and fragment analysis, which led to the birth of a healthy baby girl [96]. However, because of lack of information at the molecular level, the majority of X-linked conditions are still being carried out by sex selection.

Sex selection is not an option for certain disorders such as fragile X syndrome. It is an unusual monogenic X-linked disease where both sons and daughters could be affected when the transmitted allele comes from a carrier mother. It has been estimated that about 16% of daughters and 50% of sons are at risk of inheriting this disease (http://www.ncbi.nlm.nih.gov/omim/). This disease is caused by the expansion of unstable trinucleotide repeat CGG present at the 5' end of the *FMR-1* gene. This trinucleotide repeat is polymorphic in the population. The normal allele may vary from 6 to 54 repeats, whereas full mutation may have more than 200 repeats [63]. The heterozygosity of this repeat in the population was exploited to develop PGD for fraxile X syndrome [97]. Preimplantation diagnosis of two informative couples resulted in a pregnancy in one of the patients, and the fetus was diagnosed as unaffected when tested by prenatal diagnosis.

VIII.   MISDIAGNOSIS CONTRIBUTING FACTORS

A.   Contamination

One of the potential problems for PGD is contamination. Compared to routine PCR protocol, single-cell amplification requires a large number of PCR cycles to obtain sufficient product for analysis. Unfortunately, this process also amplifies any exogenous DNA that may have been incorporated during handling the sample. Contamination could come from sperm, cumulus cells, operator, or exogenous DNA through reagents and the equipment used. Stringent laboratory practices should be carried out in any laboratory performing single-cell PCR for diagnostic purposes. Some of the precautions taken to reduce contamination during IVF and biopsy procedures are (1) performing intracytoplasmic sperm injection (ICSI) to reduce contamination from sperm sticking to the zona pellucida, (2) removal of all cumulus cells from the egg, and (3) washing of biopsied cell in several drops of sterile medium before transferring it to the PCR tube.

In addition to taking precautions for preventing contamination, several studies show that inclusion of STR markers in the test may reduce the possibility of misdiagnosis. The high degree of heterozygosity produced by many STRs make these markers highly suitable for

DNA fingerprinting. If parental STR profiles are analyzed prior to PGD, then samples contaminated with extrinsic DNA can be easily identified during PGD and discarded.

B. Allele Drop-Out

Aside from DNA contamination, ADO is perhaps the single most serious problem associated with single-cell PCR. The reason underlying the cause of failure to amplify one of the alleles is still not fully understood. It has been suggested that it may be due to suboptimal PCR conditions [14,98–101]. Another potential difficulty is chromosomal mosaicism. This is observed because two or more cells from the same embryo may have different chromosome complements. For genetic analysis, ADO and chromosomal mosaicism will not cause serious misdiagnosis in an autosomal-recessive disorder (involving one mutation) because at least one of the two mutated alleles will be detected within an affected homozygous embryo. A heterozygous carrier could be misdiagnosed as either normal or affected. Fortunately, the only consequence of this would be the failure to identify some carrier embryos for transfer. However, in autosomal-dominant conditions or in autosomal-recessive compound heterozygotes, failure to amplify the mutant allele (PCR failure or loss of the chromosome) would lead to transfer of an affected embryo [102].

Advancements in single-cell genetic analysis have prompted different groups to address the problem of ADO and chromosomal mosaicism. In reports that examined ADO, the frequency of amplification failure has varied. Allele drop-out frequencies have been quoted as ranging from 0.8 to 36% for cystic fibrosis genetic analysis [98,100, 101,103–107]. One of the approaches to detect ADO in a sample is incorporation of a linked polymorphism in the PCR assay. By using this approach, it is possible to decrease the risk of misdiagnosis due to ADO and the inadvertent sampling of a haploid cell. The benefit of co-amplification of a linked polymorphic marker along with the specific mutation has been shown in several studies, including those for APC [94], thalassemia [71,107], and cystic fibrosis [107].

The increased sensitivity of fluorescent PCR has been attributed to low ADO rate in some of the studies performed for diagnostic tests.

Findlay and co-workers [83] reported a low ADO rate (~4%) due to an ability to distinguish true ADO from preferential amplification of one allele. Similarly, Sermon and co-workers [80] were able to demonstrate a reduction in ADO rates as a consequence of using fluorescent PCR. Like conventional PCR, a range of ADO rates has been reported using fluorescent PCR [108,109], thus emphasizing the importance of careful PCR standardization.

One alternative approach put forward to reduce ADO and amplification failure rates is the use of reverse transcription-polymerase chain reaction (RT-PCR). Compared to single-cell DNA analysis, where diagnosis is based on one allele each in a heterozygous blastomere, there may be more abundant mRNA transcripts for the targeted gene. Eldadah and colleagues [110] used this approach successfully to treat a couple at risk of Marfan's syndrome. Although this methodology could be useful for genes that are expressed at the cleavage stage, the use of RT-PCR as a diagnostic tool for PGD requires careful evaluation. Failure of amplification has been reported for a significant proportion of embryonic transcripts at the cleavage stage of development, and it was attributed to the persistence of oocyte-derived transcripts [111].

IX. CONCLUSIONS

Over the last 10 years, genetic diagnosis at the single-cell level has improved tremendously. Increased understanding of early embryo development and advances made with molecular technology have helped to develop better and more accurate tests for both chromosome analysis and single-gene defects. From the available data, the pregnancy rate in this group of patients is similar to that of infertile patients treated by IVF. Relatively low pregnancy rates in this group of mostly fertile patients may be due to many factors. The presence of a high rate of chromosomal mosaicism observed in the cleavage stage of development may have an effect on embryonic development and their survival. Also the fact that the embryo selection for transfer in PGD cycles is not based on the morphology, as is done in routine IVF, but is based on results from genetic analysis thus limiting morphologically good quality embryos for transfer. Future improvement of the overall IVF success rate combined with further progress in diagnostic tools for genetic analysis of the embryonic cell will help increase the success rates for PGD patients.

REFERENCES

1. Handyside AH, Kontogianni EH, Hardy K, Winston RM. Pregnancies from biopsied human preimplantation embryos sexed by Y-specific DNA amplification. Nature 1990; 344:768–770.
2. Verlinsky Y, Ginsberg N, Lifchez A, Valle J, Moise J, Strom CM. Analysis of the first polar body: preconception genetic diagnosis. Hum Reprod 1990; 5:826–829.
3. Verlinsky Y, Cieslak J, Ivakhnenko V, Lifchez A, Strom C, Kuliev A. Birth of healthy children after preimplantation diagnosis of common aneuploidies by polar body fluorescent in situ hybridization analysis. Preimplantation Genetic Group. Fertil Steril 1996; 66:126–129.
4. Ao A, Handyside AH. Cleavage stage human embryo biopsy. Hum Reprod Update 1995; 1:3–4.
5. Hardy K, Martin KL, Leese HJ, Winston RM, Handyside AH. Human preimplantation development in vitro is not adversely affected by biopsy at the 8-cell stage. Hum Reprod 1990; 5:708–714.
6. Dokras A, Sargent IL, Ross C, Gardner RL, Barlow DH. Trophectoderm biopsy in human blastocysts. Hum Reprod 1990; 5:821–825.
7. Muggleton Harris AL, Glazier AM, Pickering SJ. Biopsy of the human blastocyst and polymerase chain reaction (PCR) amplification of the beta-globin gene and a dinucleotide repeat motif from 2-6 trophectoderm cells. Hum Reprod 1993; 8:2197–2205.
8. Pickering SJ, Muggleton Harris AL. Reliability and accuracy of polymerase chain reaction amplification of two unique target sequences from biopsies of cleavage-stage and blastocyst-stage human embryos. Hum Reprod 1995; 10:1021–1029.
9. Veiga A, Sandalinas M, Benkhalifa M, Boada M, Carrera M, Santalo J, Barri PN, Menezo Y. Laser blastocyst biopsy for preimplantation diagnosis in the human. Zygote 1997; 5:351–354.
10. Gardner DK, Schoolcraft WB, Wagley L, Schlenker T, Stevens J, Hesla J. A prospective randomized trial of blastocyst culture and transfer in in-vitro fertilization [see comments]. Hum Reprod 1998; 13:3434–3440.

11. Gardner DK, Vella P, Lane M, Wagley L, Schlenker T, Schoolcraft WB. Culture and transfer of human blastocysts increases implantation rates and reduces the need for multiple embryo transfers. Fertil Steril 1998; 69:84–88.

12. McKusick VA. Mendelian inheritance in man. A catalog of human genes and genetic disorders. Baltimore: Johns Hopkins University Press, 1998.

13. Handyside AH, Delhanty JDA. Cleavage stage biopsy of human embryos and diagnosis of X-linked recessive disease. In: Edwards RG, ed. Preimplantation Diagnosis of Human Genetic Disease. Cambridge, UK: Cambridge University Press, 1993:239–270.

14. Kontogianni EH, Griffin DK, Handyside AH. Identifying the sex of human preimplantation embryos in X-linked disease: amplification efficiency of a Y-specific alphoid repeat from single blastomeres with two lysis protocols. J Assist Reprod Genet 1996; 13:125–132.

15. Chong SS, Kristjansson K, Cota J, Handyside AH, Hughes MR. Preimplantation prevention of X-linked disease: reliable and rapid sex determination of single human cells by restriction analysis of simultaneously amplified ZFX and ZFY sequences. Hum Mol Genet 1993; 2:1187–1191.

16. Nakagome Y, Seki S, Nagafuchi S, Nakahori Y, Sato K. Absence of fetal cells in maternal circulation at a level of 1 in 25,000. Am J Med Genet 1991; 40:506–508.

17. Liu J, Lissens W, Devroey P, Van Steirteghem A, Liebaers I. Amplification of X- and Y-chromosome-specific regions from single human blastomeres by polymerase chain reaction for sexing of preimplantation embryos. Hum Reprod 1994; 9:716–720.

18. Wilcox AJ, Weinberg CR, O'Connor JF, Baird DD, Schlatterer JP, Canfield RE, Armstrong EG, Nisula BC. Incidence of early loss of pregnancy. N Engl J Med 1988; 319:189–194.

19. Kline J, Stein Z. Reproductive toxicology: very early pregnancy. New York: Raven Press, 1985:251–265.

20. Eiben B, Bartels I, Bahr-Porsch S, Borgmann S, Gatz G, Gellert G, Goebel R, Hammans W, Hentemann M, Osmers R. Cytogenetic analysis of 750 spontaneous abortions with the direct-preparation method of chorionic villi and its implications for studying genetic causes of pregnancy wastage. Am J Hum Genet 1990; 47:656–663.

21. Hassold TJ. Chromosome abnormalities in human reproductive wastage. Trends Genet 1986; 2:105–110.

22. Trochet-Royer CB, Sele B, Jalbert P, Pison H, Racinet C, Bernard P. Avortements spontanes et anomalies chromosomiques parentales:

etude cytogenetique de 248 couples. Re Fr Gynecol Obstet 1981; 76: 195–199.

23. Yoon PW, Freeman SB, Sherman SL, Taft LF, Gu Y, Pettay D, Flanders WD, Khoury MJ, Hassold TJ. Advanced maternal age and the risk of Down syndrome characterized by the meiotic stage of chromosomal error: a population-based study. Am J Hum Genet 1996; 58:628–633.

24. Bongso A, Chye NS, Ratnam S, Sathananthan H, Wong PC. Chromosome anomalies in human oocytes failing to fertilize after insemination in vitro. Hum Reprod 1988; 3:645–649.

25. Martin RH, MaHadevan MM, Taylor PJ, Hildebrand K, Long-Simpson L, Peterson D, Yamamoto J, Fleetham J. Chromosomal analysis of unfertilized human oocytes. J Reprod Fertil 1986; 78:673–678.

26. Pellestor F, Sele B. Assessment of aneuploidy in the human female by using cytogenetics of IVF failures. Am J Hum Genet 1988; 42:274–283.

27. Plachot M, Junca AM, Mandelbaum J, de Grouchy J, Salat Baroux J, Cohen J. Chromosome investigations in early life. II. Human preimplantation embryos. Hum Reprod 1987; 2:29–35.

28. Van Blerkom J, Henry G. Cytogenetic analysis of living human oocytes: cellular basis and developmental consequences of perturbations in chromosomal organization and complement. Hum Reprod 1988; 3: 777–790.

29. Angell RR, Aitken RJ, van Look PF, Lumsden MA, Templeton AA. Chromosome abnormalities in human embryos after in vitro fertilization. Nature 1983; 303:336–338.

30. Angell RR, Templeton AA, Aitken RJ. Chromosome studies in human in vitro fertilization. Hum Genet 1986; 72:333–339.

31. Plachot M, Mandelbaum J, Junca AM, de Grouchy J, Cohen J, Salat Baroux J, Da Lage C. Morphologic cytologic and cytogenetic studies of human embryos obtained by IVF. In: Ratnam SS, Teon ES, eds. In-vitro fertilization: Proceedings of the 12th World Congress on Fertility and Sterility. Lancs, England: Parthenon Publishing Group, 1986:61–65.

32. Zenzes MT, Casper RF. Cytogenetics of human oocytes, zygotes, and embryos after in vitro fertilization. Hum Genet 1992; 88:367–375.

33. Coonen E, Harper JC, Ramaekers FCS, Delhanty JDA, Hopman AHN, Geraedts JPM, Handyside AH. Presence of chromosomal mosaicism in abnormal human preimplantation embryos detected by fluorescent in situ hybridization (FISH). Hum Genet 1994; 54:609–615.

34. Munne S, Weier HU, Grifo J, Cohen J. Chromosome mosaicism in human embryos. Biol Reprod 1994; 51:373–379.

35. Munne S, Alikani M, Tomkin G, Grifo J, Cohen J. Embryo morphology, developmental rates, and maternal age are correlated with chromosome abnormalities. Fertil Steril 1995; 64:382–391.

36. Bahce M, Cohen J, Munne S. Preimplantation genetic diagnosis of aneuploidy: were we looking at the wrong chromosomes? J Assist Reprod Genet 1999; 16:176–181.

37. Munne S, Grifo J, Cohen J, Weier HU. Chromosome abnormalities in human arrested preimplantation embryos: a multiple-probe FISH study. Am J Hum Genet 1994; 55:150–159.

38. Harper JC, Coonen E, Handyside AH, Winston RM, Hopman AH, Delhanty JD. Mosaicism of autosomes and sex chromosomes in morphologically normal, monospermic preimplantation human embryos. Prenat Diagn 1995; 15:41–49.

39. Benkhalifa M, Menezo Y, Janny L, Pouly JL, Qumsiyeh MB. Cytogenetics of uncleaved oocytes and arrested zygotes in IVF programs. J Assist Reprod Genet 1996; 13:140–148.

40. Almeida PA, Bolton VN. The relationship between chromosomal abnormality in the human preimplantation embryo and development in vitro. Reprod Fertil Dev 1996; 8:235–241.

41. Delhanty JD, Harper JC, Ao A, Handyside AH, Winston RM. Multicolour FISH detects frequent chromosomal mosaicism and chaotic division in normal preimplantation embryos from fertile patients. Hum Genet 1997; 99:755–760.

42. Magli MC, Jones GM, Gras L, Gianaroli L, Korman I, Trounson AO. Chromosome mosaicism in day 3 aneuploid embryos that develop to morphologically normal blastocysts in vitro. Hum Reprod 2000; 15: 1781–1786.

43. Pellestor F, Girardet A, Andreo B, Lefort G, Charlieu JP. Preimplantation embryo chromosome analysis by primed in situ labeling method [published erratum appears in Fertil Steril 1997; 67:591]. Fertil Steril 1996; 66:781–786.

44. Dailey T, Dale B, Cohen J, Munne S. Association between nondisjunction and maternal age in meiosis-II human oocytes. Am J Hum Genet 1996; 59:176–184.

45. Benadiva CA, Kligman I, Munne S. Aneuploidy 16 in human embryos increases significantly with maternal age. Fertil Steril 1996; 66:248–255.

46. Tan SL, Royston P, Campbell S, Jacobs HS, Betts J, Mason B, Edwards RG. Cumulative conception and livebirth rates after in-vitro fertilisation [see comments]. Lancet 1992; 339:1390–1394.

47. Verlinsky Y, Cieslak J, Freidine M, Ivakhnenko V, Wolf G, Kovalinskaya L, White M, Lifchez A, Kaplan B, Moise J. Pregnancies following pre-conception diagnosis of common aneuploidies by fluorescent in-situ hybridization. Hum Reprod 1995; 10:1923-1927.
48. Verlinsky Y, Kuliev A. Preimplantation diagnosis of common aneuploidies in infertile couples of advanced maternal age. Hum Reprod 1996; 11:2076-2077.
49. Gianaroli L, Magli MC, Ferraretti AP, Munne S. Preimplantation diagnosis for aneuploidies in patients undergoing in vitro fertilization with a poor prognosis: identification of the categories for which it should be proposed. Fertil Steril 1999; 72:837-844.
50. Munne S, Magli C, Cohen J, Morton P, Sadowy S, Gianaroli L, Tucker M, Marquez C, Sable D, Ferraretti AP, Massey JB, Scott R. Positive outcome after preimplantation diagnosis of aneuploidy in human embryos. Hum Reprod 1999; 14:2191-2199.
51. Verlinsky Y, Cieslak J, Ivakhnenko V, Evsikov S, Wolf G, White M, Lifchez A, Kaplan B, Moise J, Valle J, Ginsberg N, Strom C, Kuliev A. Prevention of age-related aneuploidies by polar body testing of oocytes. J Assist Reprod Genet 1999; 16:165-169.
52. Verlinsky Y, Cieslak J, Ivakhnenko V, Evsikov S, Wolf G, White M, Lifchez A, Kaplan B, Moise J, Valle J, Ginsberg N, Strom C, Kuliev A. Preimplantation diagnosis of common aneuploidies by the first- and second-polar body FISH analysis. J Assist Reprod Genet 1998; 15: 285-289.
53. Strom CM, Strom S, Levine E, Ginsberg N, Barton J, Verlinsky Y. Obstetric outcomes in 102 pregnancies after preimplantation genetic diagnosis. Am J Obstet Gynecol 2000; 182:1629-1632.
54. Therman E, Susman B, Denniston C. The nonrandom participation of human acrocentric chromosomes in Robertsonian translocations. Ann Hum Genet 1989; 53(pt 1):49-65.
55. Munne S, Scott R, Sable D, Cohen J. First pregnancies after preconception diagnosis of translocations of maternal origin. Fertil Steril 1998; 69:675-681.
56. Munne S, Fung J, Cassel MJ, Marquez C, Weier HU. Preimplantation genetic analysis of translocations: case-specific probes for interphase cell analysis. Hum Genet 1998; 102:663-674.
57. Conn CM, Harper JC, Winston RM, Delhanty JD. Infertile couples with Robertsonian translocations: preimplantation genetic analysis of embryos reveals chaotic cleavage divisions. Hum Genet 1998; 102: 117-123.

58. Coonen E, Martini E, Dumoulin JC, Hollanders-Crombach HT, de Die-Smulders C, Geraedts JP, Hopman AH, Evers JL. Preimplantation genetic diagnosis of a reciprocal translocation t(3;11)(q27.3;q24.3) in siblings. Mol Hum Reprod 2000; 6:199–206.

59. Scriven PN, O'Mahony F, Bickerstaff H, Yeong CT, Braude P, Mackie OC. Clinical pregnancy following blastomere biopsy and PGD for a reciprocal translocation carrier: analysis of meiotic outcomes and embryo quality in two IVF cycles. Prenat Diagn 2000; 20:587–592.

60. McKusick VA. Mendelian inheritance in man. A catalog of human genes and genetic disorders. Baltimore: Johns Hopkins University Press, 1994.

61. Geraedts J, Handyside A, Harper J, Liebaers I, Sermon K, Staessen C, Thornhill A, Vanderfaeillie A, Viville S. ESHRE Preimplantation Genetic Diagnosis (PGD) Consortium: preliminary assessment of data from January 1997 to September 1998. ESHRE PGD Consortium Steering Committee. Hum Reprod 1999; 14:3138–3148.

62. Carey JC, Baty BJ, Johnson JP, Morrison T, Skolnick M, Kivlin J. The genetic aspects of neurofibromatosis. Ann NY Acad Sci 1986; 486:45–56.

63. Fu YH, Kuhl DP, Pizzuti A, Pieretti M, Sutcliffe JS, Richards S, Verkerk AJ, Holden JJ, Fenwick RGJ, Warren ST, et al. Variation of the CGG repeat at the fragile X site results in genetic instability: resolution of the Sherman paradox. Cell 1991; 67:1047–1058.

64. Sutherland GR, Haan EA, Kremer E, Lynch M, Pritchard M, Yu S, Richards RI. Hereditary unstable DNA: a new explanation for some old genetic questions? Lancet 1991; 338:289–292.

65. Yu S, Pritchard M, Kremer E, Lynch M, Nancarrow J, Baker E, Holman K, Mulley JC, Warren ST, Schlessinger D, et al. Fragile X genotype characterized by an unstable region of DNA. Science 1991; 252:1179–1181.

66. Ashley CT Jr, Warren ST. Trinucleotide repeat expansion and human disease. [Review]. Ann Rev Genet 1995; 29:703–728.

67. La Spada AR. Trinucleotide repeat instability: genetic features and molecular mechanisms. [Review]. Brain Pathol 1997; 7:943–963.

68. Handyside AH, Lesko JG, Tarin JJ, Winston RML, Hughes MR. Birth of a normal girl after in vitro fertilization and preimplantation diagnostic testing for cystic fibrosis. N Engl J Med 1992; 327:905–909.

69. Ao A, Ray P, Harper J, Lesko J, Paraschos T, Atkinson G, Soussis I, Taylor D, Handyside A, Hughes M, Winston RM. Clinical experience with preimplantation genetic diagnosis of cystic fibrosis (delta F508). Prenat Diagn 1996; 16:137–142.

70. Ao A, Handyside A, Winston RM. Preimplantation genetic diagnosis of cystic fibrosis (delta F508). Eur J Obstet Gynecol Reprod Biol 1996; 65:7–10.

71. Kuliev A, Rechitsky S, Verlinsky O, Ivakhnenko V, Evsikov S, Wolf G, Angastiniotis M, Georghiou D, Kukharenko V, Strom C, Verlinsky Y. Preimplantation diagnosis of thalassemias. J Assist Reprod Genet 1998; 15:219–225.

72. Kuliev A, Rechitsky S, Verlinsky O, Ivakhnenko V, Cieslak J, Evsikov S, Wolf G, Angastiniotis M, Kalakoutis G, Strom C, Verlinsky Y. Birth of healthy children after preimplantation diagnosis of thalassemias. J Assist Reprod Genet 1999; 16:207–211.

73. Kanavakis E, Vrettou C, Palmer G, Tzetis M, Mastrominas M, Traeger-Synodinos J. Preimplantation genetic diagnosis in 10 couples at risk for transmitting beta-thalassaemia major: clinical experience including the initiation of six singleton pregnancies. Prenat Diagn 1999; 19: 1217–1222.

74. Dreesen JC, Bras M, de Die-Smulders C, Dumoulin JC, Cobben JM, Evers JL, Smeets HJ, Geraedts JP. Preimplantation genetic diagnosis of spinal muscular dystrophy. Mol Hum Reprod 1998; 4:881–885.

75. Ansorge W, Sproat BS, Stegemann J, Schwager C. A non-radioactive automated method for DNA sequence determination. J Biochem Biophys Methods 1986; 13:315–323.

76. Schwartz LS, Tarleton J, Popovich B, Seltzer WK, Hoffman EP. Fluorescent multiplex linkage analysis and carrier detection for Duchenne/Becker muscular dystrophy. Am J Hum Genet 1992; 51:721–729.

77. Mansfield ES, Robertson JM, Lebo RV, Lucero MY, Mayrand PE, Rappaport E, Parrella T, Sartore M, Surrey S, Fortina P. Duchenne/Becker muscular dystrophy carrier detection using quantitative PCR and fluorescence-based strategies. Am J Med Genet 1993; 48:200–208.

78. Toth T, Findlay I, Nagy B, Papp Z. Accurate sizing of (CAG)n repeats causing Huntington disease by fluorescent PCR. Clin Chem 1997; 43: 2422–2423.

79. Findlay I, Matthews P, Toth T, Quirke P, Papp Z. Same day diagnosis of Down's syndrome and sex in single cells using multiplex fluorescent PCR. Mol Pathol 1998; 51:164–167.

80. Sermon K, De Vos A, Van de Velde H, Seneca S, Lissens W, Joris H, Vandervorst M, Van Steirteghem A, Liebaers I. Fluorescent PCR and automated fragment analysis for the clinical application of preimplantation genetic diagnosis of myotonic dystrophy (Steinhert's disease). Mol Hum Reprod 1998; 4:791–796.

81. Sermon K, Goosens V, Seneca S, Lissens W, De Vos A, Vandervorst M, Van Steirteghem A, Liebaers I. Preimplantation diagnosis for Huntington's disease (HD): clinical application and analysis of the HD expansion in affected embryos. Prenat Diagn 1998; 18:1427–1436.

82. Hattori M, Yoshioka K, Sakaki Y. High-sensitive fluorescent DNA sequencing and its application for detection and mass-screening of point mutations. Electrophoresis 1992; 13:560–565.

83. Findlay I, Ray P, Quirke P, Rutherford A, Lilford R. Allelic drop-out and preferential amplification in single cells and human blastomeres: implications for preimplantation diagnosis of sex and cystic fibrosis. Hum Reprod 1995; 10:1609–1618.

84. Sermon K, Lissens W, Joris H, Seneca S, Desmyttere S, Devroey P, van Steirteghem A, Liebaers I. Clinical application of preimplantation diagnosis for myotonic dystrophy. Prenat Diagn 1997; 17:925–932.

85. Cummings CJ, Zoghbi HY. Fourteen and counting: unraveling trinucleotide repeat diseases. Hum Mol Genet 2000; 9:909–916.

86. Brook JD, McCurrach ME, Harley HG, Buckler AJ, Church D, Aburatani H, Hunter K, Stanton VP, Thirion JP, Hudson T. Molecular basis of myotonic dystrophy: expansion of a trinucleotide (CTG) repeat at the 3' end of a transcript encoding a protein kinase family member. Cell 1992; 68:799–808.

87. Mahadevan M, Tsilfidis C, Sabourin L, Shutler G, Amemiya C, Jansen G, Neville C, Narang M, Barcelo J, O'Hoy K, et al. Myotonic dystrophy mutation: an unstable CTG repeat in the 3' untranslated region of the gene. Science 1992; 255:1253–1255.

88. Dean NL, Tan SL, Ao A. The development of preimplantation genetic diagnosis for myotonic dystrophy using multiplex fluorescent PCR and its clinical application. Mol Hum Reprod 2001; 7:895–901.

89. Geraedts J, Handyside A, Harper J, Liebaers I, Sermon K, Staessen C, Thornhill A, Viville S, Wilton L. ESHRE preimplantation genetic diagnosis (PGD) consortium: data collection II (May 2000). Hum Reprod 2000; 15:2673–2683.

90. Harton GL, Tsipouras P, Sisson ME, Starr KM, Mohoney BS, Fugger EF, Schulman JD, Kilpatrick MW, Levinson G, Black SH. Preimplantation genetic testing for Marfan syndrome. Mol Hum Reprod 1996; 2:713–715.

91. Blaszczyk A, Tang YX, Dietz HC, Adler A, Berkeley AS, Krey LC, Grifo JA. Preimplantation genetic diagnosis of human embryos for Marfan's syndrome. J Assist Reprod Genet 1998; 15:281–284.

92. Sermon K, Lissens W, Messiaen L, Bonduelle M, Vandervorst M, Van Steirteghem A, Liebaers I. Preimplantation genetic diagnosis of Marfan syndrome with the use of fluorescent polymerase chain reaction and the Automated Laser Fluorescence DNA Sequencer. Fertil Steril 1999; 71:163–166.

93. Whitelaw S, Northover JM, Hodgson SV. Attitudes to predictive DNA testing in familial adenomatous polyposis. J Med Genet 1996; 33:540–543.

94. Ao A, Wells D, Handyside AH, Winston RM, Delhanty JD. Preimplantation genetic diagnosis of inherited cancer: familial adenomatous polyposis coli. J Assist Reprod Genet 1998; 15:140–144.

95. Liu J, Lissens W, Van Broeckhoven C, Lofgren A, Camus M, Liebaers I, Van Steirteghem A. Normal pregnancy after preimplantation DNA diagnosis of a dystrophin gene deletion. Prenat Diagn 1995; 15:351–358.

96. Ray PF, Harper JC, Ao A, Taylor DM, Winston RM, Hughes M, Handyside AH. Successful preimplantation genetic diagnosis for sex linked Lesch-Nyhan Syndrome using specific diagnosis. Prenat Diagn 1999; 19:1237–1241.

97. Sermon K, Seneca S, Vanderfaeillie A, Lissens W, Joris H, Vandervorst M, Van Steirteghem A, Liebaers I. Preimplantation diagnosis for fragile X syndrome based on the detection of the non-expanded paternal and maternal CGG. Prenat Diagn 1999; 19:1223–1230.

98. Wu R, Cuppens H, Buyse I, Decorte R, Marynen P, Gordts S, Cassiman JJ. Co-amplification of the cystic fibrosis delta F508 mutation with the HLA DQA1 sequence in single cell PCR: implications for improved assessment of polar bodies and blastomeres in preimplantation diagnosis. Prenat Diagn 1993; 13:1111–1122.

99. Sermon K, Lissens W, Nagy ZP, Van Steirteghem A, Liebaers I. Simultaneous amplification of the two most frequent mutations of infantile Tay-Sachs disease in single blastomeres. Hum Reprod 1995; 10:2214–2217.

100. Gitlin SA, Lanzendorf SE, Gibbons WE. Polymerase chain reaction amplification specificity: incidence of allele dropout using different DNA preparation methods for heterozygous single cells. J Assist Reprod Genet 1996; 13:107–111.

101. Ray PF, Handyside AH. Increasing the denaturation temperature during the first cycles of amplification reduces allele dropout from single cells for preimplantation genetic diagnosis. Mol Hum Reprod 1996; 2:213–218.

102. Navidi W, Arnheim N. Using PCR in preimplantation genetic disease diagnosis. Hum Reprod 1991; 6:836–849.

103. Strom CM, Verlinsky Y, Milayeva S, Evsikov S, Cieslak J, Lifchez A, Valle J, Moise J, Ginsberg N, Applebaum M. Preconception genetic diagnosis of cystic fibrosis. [Letter]. Lancet 1990; 336:306–307.

104. Strom CM, Rechitsky S, Wolf G, Verlinsky Y. Reliability of polymerase chain reaction (PCR) analysis of single cells for preimplantation genetic diagnosis. J Assist Reprod Genet 1994; 11:55–62.

105. Avner R, Laufer N, Safran A, Kerem BS, Friedmann A, Mitrani Rosenbaum S. Preimplantation diagnosis of cystic fibrosis by simultaneous detection of the W1282X and delta F508 mutations. Hum Reprod 1994; 9:1676–1680.

106. Ray PF, Winston RML, Handyside AH. Elimination of allele dropout (ADO) in single cell analysis for diagnosis of cystic fibrosis (CF) (abstract). Hum Reprod 1995; 10:64.

107. Rechitsky S, Strom C, Verlinsky O, Amet T, Ivakhnenko V, Kukharenko V, Kuliev A, Verlinsky Y. Allele dropout in polar bodies and blastomeres. J Assist Reprod Genet 1998; 15:253–257.

108. Findlay I, Urquhart A, Quirke P, Sullivan K, Rutherford AJ, Lilford RJ. Simultaneous DNA 'fingerprinting,' diagnosis of sex and single-gene defect status from single cells. Hum Reprod 1995; 10:1005–1013.

109. Findlay I, Matthews P, Quirke P. Preimplantation genetic diagnosis using fluorescent polymerase chain reaction: results and future developments. J Assist Reprod Genet 1999; 16:199–206.

110. Eldadah ZA, Grifo JA, Dietz HC. Marfan syndrome as a paradigm for transcript-targeted preimplantation diagnosis of heterozygous mutations. Nat Med 1995; 1:798–803.

111. Taylor DM, Ray PF, Ao A, Winston RM, Handyside AH. Paternal transcripts for glucose-6-phosphate dehydrogenase and adenosine deaminase are first detectable in the human preimplantation embryo at the three- to four-cell stage. Mol Reprod Dev 1997; 48:442–448.

112. Xu K, Shi ZM, Veeck LL, Hughes MR, Rosenwaks Z. First unaffected pregnancy using preimplantation genetic diagnosis for sickle cell anemia. JAMA 1999; 281:1701–1706.

113. Van de Velde H, Sermon K, De Vos A, Lissens W, Joris H, Vandervorst M, Van Steirteghem A, Liebaers I. Fluorescent PCR and automated fragment analysis in preimplantation genetic diagnosis for 21-hydroxylase deficiency in congenital adrenal hyperplasia. Mol Hum Reprod 1999; 5:691–696.

114. Gibbons WE, Gitlin SA, Lanzendorf SE, Kaufmann RA, Slotnick RN,

Hodgen GD. Preimplantation genetic diagnosis for Tay-Sachs disease: successful pregnancy after pre-embryo biopsy and gene amplification by polymerase chain reaction. Fertil Steril 1995; 63:723–728.

115. De Vos A, Sermon K, Van de Velde H, Joris H, Vandervorst M, Lissens W, Mortier G, De Sutter P, Lofgren A, Van Broeckhoven C, Liebaers I, Van Steirteghem A. Pregnancy after preimplantation genetic diagnosis for Charcot-Marie-Tooth disease type 1A. Mol Hum Reprod 1998; 4:978–984.

116. De Vos A, Sermon K, Van de Velde H, Joris H, Vandervorst M, Lissens W, De Paepe A, Liebaers I, Van Steirteghem A. Two pregnancies after preimplantation genetic diagnosis for osteogenesis imperfecta type I and type IV. Hum Genet 2000; 106:605–613.

117. Verlinsky Y, Rechitsky S, Verlinsky O, Xu K, Schattman G, Masciangelo C, Ginberg N, Strom C, Rosenwaks Z, Kuliev A. Preimplantation diagnosis for p52 tumour suppressor gene mutations. Reprod Biomed Online 2001; 2:102–105.

118. Strom CM, Rechitsky S, Wolf G, Cieslak J, Kuliev A, Verlinsky Y. Preimplantation diagnosis of autosomal dominant retinitis pigmentosum using two simultaneous single cell assays for a point mutation in the rhodopsin gene. Mol Hum Reprod 1998; 4:351–355.

119. Lee SH, Kwak IP, Cha KE, Park SE, Kim NK, Cha KY. Preimplantation diagnosis of non-deletion Duchenne muscular dystrophy (DMD) by linkage polymerase chain reaction analysis. Mol Hum Reprod 1998; 4:345–349.

8

Human Oocyte Cryopreservation

Hang Yin and Roger G. Gosden
*The Jones Institute for Reproductive Medicine, Norfolk, Virginia,
U.S.A.*

Ahmad Kamal Abdul-Jalil
*McGill University and McGill University Health Centre, Montreal,
Quebec, Canada*

I. HISTORY OF EMBRYO AND OOCYTE CRYOPRESERVATION

Investigations of the cryopreservation of cells and tissues have succeeded in defining conditions for maintaining structural and functional integrity during the cooling stage, storage in liquid nitrogen ($-196°C$), and subsequent thawing. The discovery of cryoprotectants in 1949 [1] and their subsequent use in the cryopreservation of human sperm have made cryopreservation of human cells and tissues a reality [2,3].

It was not until the 1970s that attempts to preserve mammalian oocytes and embryos were first successful. Mouse embryos were successfully frozen by Whittingham et al. [4], and it was only 5 years later that mature mouse oocytes were then cryopreserved [5]. The procedure used in the cryopreservation of mouse embryos was extended to oocytes and embryos in a number of animal species with varying success rates [6–10].

In the 1980s, human embryo cryopreservation was introduced into clinical practice, and the first pregnancy was reported in 1983 [11]. The method of embryo cryopreservation described by Trounson [12] is now routinely used for cryopreservation of supernumerary embryos to avoid repeating a cycle of superstimulation treatment, and occasionally for fertility conservation for cancer patients [13]. Evidence from animal studies indicates that embryos and gametes may be stored at liquid nitrogen temperatures indefinitely without deterioration.

Human embryo freezing raises potential problems and has been controversial in practice; because of the risk of producing "orphan embryos." A male partner is not necessary in oocytes cryopreservation, as such, this strategy is sometimes more desirable. Another example is that improvements in the treatment of patients undergoing cancer therapy have resulted in more patients surviving the disease. Young patients are now frequently seeking to preserve their fertility potential before undergoing sterilizing chemotherapy or radiotherapy. As such, oocyte cryopreservation offers a number of important clinical applications in preserving female infertility:

- Circumvents the complex ethical, legal, social, and religious dilemmas that are associated with embryo cryopreservation;
- Provides the possibility for oocyte conservation prior to chemotherapy and radiotherapy;
- Offers the ability to store oocytes before destructive operations for gynecological diseases;
- Creates the potential to delay fertility in women with no medical indications and no immediate plans to conceive;
- Creates more efficient use of donated oocytes for the treatment of infertile couples, e.g., those who suffer from premature ovarian failure; and
- Is the preferred method where there is no male partner, which may be beneficial for young women who suffer from gynecological diseases or cancer of the reproductive system.

Therefore, the availability of an efficient cryopreservation protocol for freezing of human oocytes is an attractive option to preserve reproductive capability in women. Unfortunately, its applications are only suitable for young women because controlled stimulation is inappropriate for prepubertal children and the gametes of older women are often of poor quality.

II.   LIMITATIONS OF HUMAN OOCYTE CRYOPRESERVATION

Cryopreservation of human oocytes is still in its infancy and is primarily a research procedure. Despite being an attractive option to embryo cryopreservation since the first births from cryopreserved oocytes [14], there was little enthusiasm for using the technique because of low survival and fertilization rates, and only occasional pregnancy successes [15–17]. The lack of success of cryopreserved oocytes compared to embryos was due to lower post-thaw oocyte survival rates, which varied between 4 and 95% (Table 1). Recently, improved survival rates coupled with better fertilization rates obtained with intracytoplasmic sperm injection (ICSI) of thawed oocytes have resulted in several more pregnancies and births [18–26]. More recently, Fabbri et al. [27] reported an even higher survival rate (60–82%) with a modified protocol.

Several problems (to be discussed in the next section) have to be resolved before this technology can be utilized routinely in an in vitro fertilization (IVF) program. Thus, the challenge to researchers is developing the optimal protocol for storage of human unfertilized oocytes at low temperature.

III.   FUNDAMENTALS OF CRYOBIOLOGY AND ITS RELATION TO HUMAN OOCYTES CRYOPRESERVATION

The success of any cryopreservation program depends on adhering to basic principles of cryobiology. In the absence of cryoprotective agents (CPAs), most mammalian cells will not survive exposure to subzero temperatures, mainly due to two major classes of physical stresses: direct effects of reduced temperature and physical changes associated with ice formation. Chilling injury includes damage to cell structure and function arising from a sudden reduction of temperature, which is associated with changes in membrane structure and permeability, and in the cytoskeletal structure, as well as other factors in mammalian oocytes (Table 2).

Table 1 Summary of Published Reports on Cryopreservation of Mature or Immature Human Oocytes

Reference	Cryoprotectant	Freezing methods (*)	Number of oocytes with (+) or without (−) cumulus	Stage of oocytes	Post-thaw survival (%)	Oocytes fertilized (%)	Insemination method	Embryo cleavage (%)	Pregnancy/birth
12	PROH	1	6 (+)	MII	4 (67)	4 (100)	IVF	NA	No transfer
	DMSO	2	3 (+)	MII	0 (0)	NA	NA	NA	No transfer
	DMSO	4	18 (+)	MII	9 (50)	NA	NA	NA	No transfer
	DMSO	4	6 (−)	MII	4 (67)	3 (75)	IVF	0 (0)	No transfer
			16 (+)	MII	10 (63)	4 (40)	IVF	3 (75)	No transfer
16	DMSO	2	4 (+)	MII	NA	2	IVF	2 (100)	Yes/1
15	DMSO	1	144 (+)	MII	40 (28)	20 (50)	IVF	NA	Yes (2)/none
	PROH + sucrose	1	38 (+)	MII	12 (32)	9 (75)	IVF	NA	No transfer
	DMSO + sucrose	3	23 (+)	MII	1 (4)	0 (0)	IVF	NA	Yes (2)/none
74	DMSO	1	136 (+)	MII	43 (32)	25 (58)	IVF	NA	Yes/3
88	DMSO	1	50 (+)	MII	38 (76)	27 (71)	IVF	23 (85)	No transfer
71	DMSO	1	56 (+ or −)	MII	20 (36)	6 (30)	NA	NA	No transfer
	DMSO or PROH ± sucrose	1	27 (+ or −)	GV or MI	10 (37)	2 (20)	NA	NA	No transfer
17	DMSO	1	38 (NA)	MII	14 (37)	7 (50)	IVF	NA	Yes/1
49	DMSO + sucrose	4	82 (−)	MII	44 (54)	NA	NA	NA	No transfer
72	DMSO	1	48 (NA)	MII	20 (42)	7 (33)	IVF	NA	No transfer
	PROH	1	16 (NA)	MII	10 (63)	0 (0)[b]	IVF	–	No transfer
73	Glycerol	1	13 (−)	MII	8 (62)	3 (38)	IVF	0 (0)	No transfer
	DMSO	1	15 (−)	MII	11 (73)	5 (45)	IVF	1 (20)	No transfer
52	PROH + sucrose	1	33 (+)	MII	18 (55)	8 (44)	IVF	6 (75)	No transfer
	PROH + sucrose	1	30 (−)	MII	8 (27)	2 (25)	IVF	1 (50)	No transfer

29	PROH + sucrose	1	48 (+)	MII + G	23 (48)	NA	NA	NA	No transfer
86	PROH + sucrose	1	131 (−)	V MII	91 (69)	NA	NA	NA	No transfer
77	PROH + sucrose	1	134 (−)	MII	55 (41)	25 (46)	IVF	NA	No transfer
	PROH	1	77 (+)	GV	12 (16)	NA	NA	—	—
78	PROH + sucrose	1	67 (+)	GV	22 (43)	NA	NA	—	—
61	PROH + sucrose	1	123 (+)	GV	72 (59)	30/52 (58)	IVF	1 (3.3)	No transfer
94	PROH + sucrose	1	26 (−)	MII	18 (69)	9 (50)	IVF	9 (100)	No transfer
	PROH + sucrose	1	20 (−)	MII	19 (95)	7 (27)	ICSI	7 (100)	No transfer
	DMSO, PROH; EG, acetamide	4	20 (−)	MII	13 (65)	9 (45)	IVF	0 (0)	No transfer
110	PROH + sucrose	1	90 (NA)	MII	29 (32)	15 (52)	IVF	10 (15)	Yes/none
91	PROH + sucrose	1	220 (−)	MII	37 (34)	1 (3)	IVF	0 (0)	No transfer
89	PROH + sucrose	1	81 (−)	MII	37 (34)	16 (43)	ICSI	16 (100)	No transfer
18	PROH + sucrose	1	12 (−)	MII	20 (25)	13 (65)	ICSI	13 (100)	Yes (3)/none
20	PROH + sucrose	1	10 (+)	MII	4 (33)	2 (50)	ICSI	1 (50)	Yes/1[a]
21	PROH + sucrose	1	129 (NA)	MII	3 (30)	2 (67)	ICSI	2 (100)	Yes/1
75	PROH + sucrose	1	NA (+)	MII	66 (51)	34 (51)	ICSI	32 (94)	Yes/3
			NA (−)	MII	(54)	(44)	ICSI	(75)	Yes (6)/1+
				MII	(27)	(25)	ICSI	(50)	NA (?)
19	PROH	1	709 (−)	MII	396 (56)	248 (63)	ICSI	223 (90)	Yes (9)/6
87	PROH + sucrose	1	9 (−)	MII	8 (89)	8 (100)	ICSI	5 (63)	Yes/marriage
23	PROH + sucrose	1	241 (−)	MII	75 (31)	38 (51)	ICSI	NA	Yes (5)/2
76	PROH + sucrose	1	16 (−)	GV	7 (44)	3 (43)	ICSI	3 (100)	Yes/1
13	PROH + sucrose	1	13 (−)	GV	3 (23)	2/2 (100)	ICSI	2 (100)	Yes/1
92	PROH + sucrose	1	54 (NA)	GV	42 (78)	NA	ICSI	NA	Yes/none
	PROH + sucrose	1	7 (NA)	MII	3 (43)	1 (33)	ICSI	1 (100)	Yes/marriage
24	PROH + sucrose	1	14 (NA)	MII	3 (21)	NA	NA	NA	No transfer
	PROH + sucrose	1	16 (NA)	MII	11 (69)	NA	NA	NA	No transfer

Table 1 Continued

Reference	Cryoprotectant	Freezing methods (*)	Number of oocytes with (+) or without (−) cumulus	Stage of oocytes	Post-thaw survival (%)	Oocytes fertilized (%)	Insemination method	Embryo cleavage (%)	Pregnancy/birth
53	EG + sucrose	4	37 (NA)	MII	34 (92)	22 (65)	ICSI	17 (77)	Yes/NA
54	EG + sucrose	4	17 (−)	MII	11 (65)	5 (45)	ICSI	3 (60)	Yes/1
47	PROH + sucrose	1	15 (−)	MII	11 (73)	5 (45)	ICSI	5 (100)	Yes/1[b]
93	PROH + sucrose	1	10 (−)	MII	7 (70)	5 (71)	ICSI	3 (60)	Yes/2[c]
24	PROH + sucrose	1	120 (NA)	MII	68 (57)	54 (79)	ICSI	NA	Yes (7)/4 + ?
26	PROH + sucrose	1	11 (−)	MII	9 (82)	7 (78)	ICSI	6 (86)	Yes/no
99	EG + sucrose	4	17 (+)	MII	11 (65)	6/9 (67)	ICSI	5 (83)	No transfer
70	EG + sucrose	4	90 (+)	MII	57 (63)	39 (68)	ICSI	35 (89)	Yes/2 + ?
109	PROH + sucrose	1	85 (+)	MII	51 (60)	39 (76)	ICSI	32 (82)	No transfer
27	PROH + sucrose	1	1502 (+ or −)	MII	765 (54)	365/632 (58)	ICSI	332 (91)	No transfer

* 1 = Slow freezing–rapid thawing; 2 = slow freezing/slow thawing; 3 = ultra-rapid freezing; 4 = vitification; NA = not available; PROH = 1,2-propanediol; DMSO = dimethysulfoxide; EG = ethylene glycol; ICSI = intracytoplasmic sperm injection.
[a] First birth of ICSI of cryopreserved oocytes.
[b] First birth with testicular sperm.
[c] First birth with epididymal sperm.

Table 2 Susceptible Factors in Mammalian Oocytes Damaged
by Cooling and Cryopreservation

Factors	Type of damage
Membrane	Rupture, leakage, fusion
Actin	No extrusion of the second polar body, destroy the union of sperm and egg nuclei after fertilization and inhibit embryo cleavage
Spindles	Depolymerization of microtubules and straying of chromosomes
Nuclear/Chromosomes	Aneuploidy, digyny (failure to extrude polar body), polyploidy, apoptosis, parthogenesis
Cortical granules	Premature release and zone pellucida hardening
Cytoplasmic organelles	Damage or loss function of mitochondria, Golgi body, endoplasmic reticulum and lysosome, affect structural and functional integrity of oocytes
Proteins	Dehydration and loss of function
Lipids	Cold sensitive and peroxidation

Source: Modified from Ref. 111.

Despite these considerable difficulties, several effective protocols
for cryopreservation of oocytes of the mouse [6,28], the cow [9] and
other species have been developed. Unfortunately, these mammalian
protocols are not ideal for human oocytes because of differences in
size, cellular properties, sensitivity to cooling, and permeability to
cryoprotectants. The human oocyte is the largest cell in the body,
which is a critical parameter because of the low surface-to-volume ratio.
More importantly, it was demonstrated that human oocytes behave dif-
ferently from oocytes of animal models. A successful human oocyte
cryopreservation protocol applied to mouse oocytes displayed only 1%
survival after 24 hr freeze-thaw; thus the mouse model should not be
relied on for investigations of human oocyte freezing [29].

The major cause of oocyte injury during freezing and thawing is
the formation of intracellular ice crystals [30], which is invariably le-
thal. The structures that are susceptible to damage during freeze-thaw
of human oocytes are the zona pellucida, cortical granules, the meiotic

spindle in metaphase oocytes, and microfilaments in ooplasm and the cytoplasmic organelles. In addition, parthenogenetic activation (spontaneous cleavage of the oocyte without fertilization by a spermatozoa) is another major problem in freeze–thaw oocytes, which can be introduced by thermal shock or chemical toxicity, such as from cryoprotectants. However, the mechanism by which this activation is introduced is less known, although elevated intracellular calcium ions are believed to be involved [31,32].

During fertilization of human oocytes, one of the mechanisms preventing polyspermy is the cortical granule reaction. The movement of cortical granules toward the perivitelline space and the exocytosis of their contents containing hydrolytic enzymes, other proteins, and sugars leads to a change of zona pellucida structure and the inactivation of sperm receptors [33]. In the presence of cryoprotectants, early exocytosis of cortical granules could trigger premature zona hardening, thus causing a significant reduction in fertilization rates [34,35]. On the other hand, low temperature could compromise the zona reaction by reducing the number of cortical granules [36], leading to polyspermy.

More importantly, the meiotic spindle of mature (metaphase II) oocytes is susceptible to damage during the freeze–thaw procedure. The meiotic spindles are reported to be highly sensitive to temperature changes [37,38]. Cooling causes the depolymerization of microtubules [39,40], leading to separate binding of chromosomes on the spindle apparatus during the cell division. This could result in aneuploidy in freeze–thaw oocytes after the extrusion of the second polar body [41,42]. Moreover, abnormal distribution of microfilaments was observed in bovine oocytes after thawing [43], leading to the improper rotation of spindle apparatus and extrusion of the polar body, which may lead to digynic oocytes [44,45]. However, the spindle in mouse oocytes has a larger tolerance to lower temperature and has the capacity to reverse the disruption of the meiotic spindle caused in the freeze–thaw procedure and to repolymerize in an appropriate manner [46].

In addition, in our recent study, mouse metaphase II oocytes were frozen using a slow freezing and rapid thawing protocol with 1.5 M ethylene glycol as the CPA. Meiotic spindles did not show major damage compared to the control group (97 vs. 91% with normal morphol-

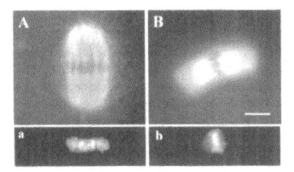

Figure 1 Spindle formation and chromosome behavior in fresh isolated (A,a) or freeze–thaw (B,b) mouse metaphase II oocytes. Oocytes show a barrel-shaped bipolar spindle with chromosomes well aligned at the equator plate. Bar = 10 μm. (a,b): 4′,6-Diamidino-2-phenylindole (DAPI) stained chromosomes. (A,B): antitubulin immunofluorescence with fluorescein isothiocyanate FITC.

ogy, Fig. 1). Therefore, it is of interest to study the factors involved in protecting the meiotic spindle in mouse oocytes from cryoinjury.

IV. CRYOPRESERVATION OF HUMAN OOCYTES

A. Cryoprotectant Agent (Permeating and Nonpermeating)

Exposing cells to low temperatures without the addition of protective compounds results in intracellular ice formation, leading to cell death. However, the use of cryoprotectants in freezing is important in several ways. First, they lower the freezing point, until very low temperatures are reached, thus aiding further dehydration of the oocytes. Second, cryoprotectants interact with membranes as they change from the pliable to rigid state during cooling. Among the technical variables, cryoprotectants are believed to play a major role in oocyte survival [47] because they reduce electrolyte concentration in the unfrozen medium, thus reducing the amount of water that crystallizes.

There are two types of cryoprotectants—permeating substances and nonpermeating substances. Permeating cryoprotectants (e.g., glycerol, 1,2-propanediol [PROH], dimethylsulfoxide [DMSO], and ethylene glycol [EG]) are fairly small molecules that permeate cell membranes easily. Concentrations of permeating cryoprotectants, are usually many times higher than any other component of the cryopreservation medium; 1–2 M for slow freezing and at least 3–4 M for ultrarapid freezing [48]. Cryoprotectants enter the cells by diffusion and intracellular water leaves the cell by osmosis to dilute the increasing concentration of solutes as extracellular ice forms. Thus shrinkage of the oocyte occurs [48], and continues until osmotic equilibrium is reached.

Nonpermeating substances (e.g., sucrose) are usually large molecules and they do not permeate the cell membrane. This kind of cryoprotectant used together with standard permeating cryoprotectants results in increased dehydration and intracellular concentration of permeating cryoprotectant before freezing [49,50]. In a large study of approximately 900 human oocytes, Fabbri et al. [27] showed that freezing oocytes using a solution of 1.5 M PROH and 0.3 mol/L sucrose enhanced oocyte survival rates when compared to lower sucrose concentration, suggesting that insufficient dehydration is fatal. A longer exposure time (10.5–15 min) to the cryoprotective solution positively affects the oocyte survival rate. Tucker et al. [23] further reiterated that the key to cryosurvival was the effective passage of cryoprotectant across the cell membrane through an extended exposure time plus the use of serum.

In oocyte cryopreservation, many early investigators used DMSO with limited success [12,14–16]. Others utilized PROH because it is seen to be less toxic than DMSO, and has been an excellent cryoprotectant for freezing of cleaved embryos and oocytes [29,51]. However, no controlled trial has ever been undertaken. The use of PROH and sucrose in oocyte cryopreservation gave good survival rates [29,52]. Recently, [53] and Kuleshova et al. [54] successfully utilized EG and sucrose in vitrification of human oocytes. In addition, Pensis et al. [49] performed vitrification of human oocytes and showed that increased sucrose concentration (e.g., 0.2 M with DMSO) resulted in a better survival rate.

B. Cryopreservation Program

Cryopreservation protocols for human oocytes can be broadly classified as "slow" or "rapid," based on the rate of cooling and concentration of cryoprotectants. Basically, the ultimate aim is to protect the oocytes from chilling injury, intracellular ice formation, dehydration, and toxic effects of cryoprotectants.

Slow Freezing/Rapid Thawing

Slow freezing/rapid thawing techniques are commonly used for preserving human oocytes. The slow freezing protocol performed using a controlled freezing apparatus reduces the amount of water within the cells to minimize intracellular ice formation. This is achieved by placing the cells in a solution containing 10–11% (v/v) penetrating cryoprotectant (approximately 1.5 M), and cooling at a controlled cooling rate, usually, for example, from 22 to −4.5 to −8°C at a rate of 2°C/min. The lower the temperature, the more water molecules that freeze, leaving solute in aqueous phase to increase concentration, which draws water out of the cells osmotically. This can damage the cells because of the so-called solution effect of cooling [55]. Therefore, the success of slow cooling depends on achieving the optimal balance between the rate at which water can leave a cell and the rate at which it is converted into ice. Furthermore, the freezing point of the remaining solution is lowered, which is known as super-cooling. Ice nucleation is initiated (seeding) manually at a temperature between −4.5 and −8°C to minimize possible deleterious effects due to the release of latent heat of crystallization at a super-cooling temperature, which is necessary for cell survival [4,56]. When human oocytes were preserved in 1.5 M PROH solution, the seeding temperature at −4.5°C gave the most effective survival rate [57]. Slow freezing has proven to be a valuable tool in human embryo cryopreservation [11]. After the manual seeding (ice nucleation) is performed, the cells are cooled at a rate of 0.2–0.3°C/min to −30°C, followed by rapid cooling of 10–30°C/min to −150°C. The thawing is usually rapid at ∼100°C/min. The cryoprotectant is removed by transferring the oocytes stepwise in decreasing concentrations of cryoprotectant, which can protect oocytes from swelling and lysis. Sugar is usually added to these dilutions to reduce the risk of damage by water entering the cell too rapidly [48]. This technique is successful in oocyte and embryo freezing in various animals and in human embryos [27,58–61], but a corresponding slow freezing protocol for optimal cryopreservation of human oocytes has yet to be achieved.

Vitrification

Alternatively, rapid freezing such as vitrification is designed to eliminate the need for expensive freezing equipment. It involves the use of high concentration of cryoprotectant with ultrarapid freezing rate, usually at a cooling rate of 10,000°C/min. It is potentially less damaging than slow freezing because it avoids the formation of intracellular ice during equilibrium cooling and warming [54]. Recent reports in both the domestic cattle industry and mouse have demonstrated that vitrification of oocytes resulted in better survival rates than slow freezing [62–64]. Cells are vitrified using high concentrations of penetrating cryoprotectants; increased viscosity occurs to the point that the solution solidifies into a glasslike state, thus avoiding ice crystal formation and subsequent damaging osmotic effects [62]. Recent research has focused on vitrification of human oocytes, which contain large volumes of water in the ooplasm [8,9,49]. However, limitations of vitrification of human oocytes are evident, because high cryoprotectant concentrations are toxic to oocytes, thus requiring brief equilibration steps or equilibration at reduced temperatures [48,54,65]. EG-based vitrification solution can be quite toxic to mouse embryo cells at temperatures of 25°C or higher and prolonged exposure of 2 min or more [66]. Exposing mouse oocytes to the vitrification solution for 15 sec was found to be optimal, resulting in high survival rates (77–89%) and good development of hatching blastocysts (31.8%) [67]. Alternative cryoprotectants are sugar, and other polymers, Ficol, serum, etc., which are less toxic [66,68,69]. Vitrified oocytes are also thawed in a stepwise manner of decreasing concentrations of the cryoprotectant at low temperatures, to avoid the toxic effects of cryoprotectants. So far, good survival, fertilization rates, embryo cleavage, and even live births have been demonstrated by vitrification in a number of human IVF centers [54,70].

The potential benefits of vitrification for human oocytes needs to be further explored.

C. Selection of Oocytes for Cryopreservation

Oocytes recovered from patients can be frozen in relatively short periods of time after oocyte collection. Which stage of the human oocyte would be able to provide high survival rates, good fertilization rate, and subsequent cleavage even to the blastocyst stage in an efficient cryopreservation program? Which factors determine the successful selection of oocytes?

Mature (Metaphase II) Oocytes

Early investigators achieved sporadic success with births from cryopreserved mature oocytes that were made available from patients undergoing treatment in a gonadotropin-stimulated IVF program [14,16]. However, there was a lack of confidence in using the technique due to low survival rates [17,71], poor fertilization [72,73], and a high incidence of polyploidy [15]. It was shown that exposure of mouse [39] and human [40] oocytes to reduction in temperatures induced depolymerization of the spindle tubulin, giving the appearance of a disrupted or disorganized spindle, and in some cases its complete absence [38]. Gook et al. [29] observed a similar proportion of abnormal spindles when human oocytes were exposed to cryoprotectants at room temperature. Thus, a cryopreservation protocol which could avoid these potential problems associated with mature oocytes, such as disruption of the meiotic spindle and disorganization of the chromosomes (leading to an increase in the rate of aneuploidy and subsequent low fertilization), needs to be explored by researchers.

However, all the early births from cryopreserved oocytes were from mature metaphase II (MII) oocytes [14,16,17]. This observation was later confirmed by Al-Hasani et al. [15] and Diedrich et al. [74], where cryopreserved mature oocytes resulted in a higher percentage of intact oocyte compared to intermediate-mature (metaphase I) or immature (germinal veside [GV]) oocytes. These were achieved using DMSO in a slow-freezing cryopreservation protocol [14–17]. This was despite the fact that mature oocytes are particularly susceptible to freeze–thaw damage due to their size and complexity, particularly to the meiotic spindle, which was highlighted in reports of increased post-thaw aneuploidy in the mouse model [41]. Fertilization of surviving human oocytes was similar to standard IVF protocols.

Subsequently, the use of PROH and sucrose in a similar cryopreservation protocol resulted in consistently good survival rates [21,29,75] and several births [18,20,21,23,76]. Gook et al. [77] showed that surviving oocytes had normal karyotypes and an absence of stray chromosomes, even in oocytes that had abnormal fertilization. Because PROH is widely regarded to be less toxic and more permeable than DMSO, they concluded that cryopreservation with PROH maintained sufficient oocyte integrity for normal fertilization (approximately equal to IVF rates of fresh oocytes), thus showing that in the surviving oocytes, there is minimal damage to the zona pellucida, plasma membrane, cytoskeleton, and cortical granules. In fact, however, a controlled trial to compare these substances has never been performed.

Immature (Germinal Vesicle) Oocytes

Cryopreservation of immature (GV) oocytes is an alternative approach to storage of human oocytes. In these oocytes, meiosis is arrested at the diplotene stage and chromosomes are within the membrane-bound nucleus, and are able to better survive the cryopreservation procedure and mature after thawing [78,79]. In theory, this approach may avoid cryoinjury to the meiotic spindle and may reduce the frequency of chromosomal disturbances in the freeze–thaw oocyte.

In the mouse, it was observed that freeze–thaw immature oocytes were capable of re-establishing an apparently normal nucleus and cytoplasm, and further culture of these oocytes lead to high maturity rates. These oocytes can be fertilized and are capable of undergoing the normal process of preimplantation and embryogenesis [80–83]. In the patients undergoing stimulated IVF cycles, immature oocytes may be recovered during development of multiple follicles and without exposing them to human chorionic gonadatropin (HCG). These recovered GV oocytes may be cryopreserved [84]. Despite the potential benefits of immature human oocytes cryopreservation, it is yet undetermined whether this optimism is justified [23,76].

Presence or Absence of Cumulus Cells

The effect of the presence or removal of the cumulus oophorus prior to oocyte cryopreservation has been little studied and reports have been conflicting. Early reports of human oocyte cryopreservation showed good survival rates with partial cumulus removal [14,16]. These were further supported by recent reports highlighting increased survival rates from cryopreserved cumulus-intact oocytes [52,75]. Conversely, Gook et al. [29] found that oocytes surrounded by a complete cumulus and corona mass had significantly reduced survival rates compared to oocytes that had the cumulus mass reduced prior to freezing. It was suggested that there was a difference in the rate of dehydration in the presence of cumulus cells. Also, the cumulus corona complex may form a more rigid structure, limiting the distortion of the oocyte shape when in the cryopreservation medium [85]. The hypothesis is that oocytes and cumulus cells are two types of cells with different morphological and biophysiological characteristics, thus different permeability to cryoprotectant and cellular dehydration during chemical equilibration [29]. Fabbri et al. [75] reiterated that a better oocyte survival rate was obtained in oocytes with partially removed cumulus, but a later report from the same group found that the cumulus complex did not significantly improve oocyte survival [27,86]. This was in agreement with the experience of Mandelbaum et al. [71].

The survival rates of cryopreserving oocytes with cumulus intact or partially dissected varied from 2 to 80% [14–16]. In addition, Hunter et al. [73] achieved good post-thaw survival rates for denuded oocytes. A few comparative cryopreservation studies involving the role of cumulus in oocyte survival showed contradictory outcomes [29,52,75]. Therefore, the effect of cumulus oophorus in oocyte cryopreservation and its corresponding role have to be further investigated.

D. Timing of Oocyte Freezing

Early investigators cryopreserved oocytes between 2 and 6 hr post-oocyte recovery [12,15] with reasonably good survival rates. Good survival rates were obtained even when the oocytes were frozen as late as 8 hr post-collection [77,87]. However, in an earlier report, Gook et al. [29] showed that there was no difference in initial survival rates in oocytes incubated on day 0, 1, or ≥2 days. Re-examination of the surviving oocytes 24 hr post-thaw revealed reduction in survival rates, with a significant decrease in rates when comparing day 0 and day 1 rates. It was suggested that with increased age, oocytes are more sensitive to subzero temperatures, or the ionic changes and dehydration during cryopreservation. Furthermore, freezing aged oocytes produced a decrease in normal fertilization rate and increased polyploidy [77]. Cryopreserved oocytes that survived but did not fertilize showed absent or abnormal spindles. No scattering of chromosomes was observed in the cytoplasm, even in those with abnormal spindles where the chromosomes were in clumps.

So far, most programs perform oocyte cryopreservation 2–8 hr after oocyte recovery [16,18,77,88]. Others have performed oocyte cryopreservation 12 hr [26] post-collection due to circumstances, or as long as 24 hr [23] post-collection for convenience.

V. ACHIEVEMENTS OF CRYOPRESERVATION OF HUMAN OOCYTES

The efficiency of oocyte cryopreservation is seriously deficient compared with embryo cryopreservation. Early results for survival, fertilization, and cleavage have been disappointing, leading to only sporadic pregnancies over the last 10 years. However, encouraging achievements have been made in increasing the survival rates, fertilization of oocytes, embryo cleavage rates, and pregnancy/live birth rates.

A. Survival Rate

Oocytes were classified as surviving the freeze–thaw procedure only if (1) the zona pellucida and cytoplasmic membrane were intact; and (2) the perivitelline space was clear and normal in size, and there was no cytoplasmic leakage and/or oocyte shrinkage [75].

Early investigators obtained an average survival rate of 37% using DMSO in cryopreservation of human oocytes [15,74,88]. Subsequently, an average of 50% oocyte survival rate has been obtained with PROH as the cryoprotectant [19,21–23,89], and recently, Porcu [86] and colleagues [90] reported a mean survival rate of 58–60% in a large series of freeze–thaw oocytes, which probably represents the highest efficiency, at present, for this technique.

B. Fertilization and Cleavage Rates

Fertilization rates obtained with freeze/thaw oocytes is extremely variable, ranging from 3% [91] to 71% [88], with 46% being the average fertilization rate observed in a large study [86]. Many programs utilized PROH and insemination by ICSI [61,89,91]. Fertilization rates by ICSI ranged from 25% to 100%; the report by Porcu [47] reporting average rates of 60%.

C. Pregnancy/Implantation rate/Live-Birth Rate

Mandelbaum and colleagues [13] reviewed data on cryopreservation of mature human oocytes (up to 1994) and reported a live birth rate of 1% (birth of four babies from 383 thawed oocytes). In a total of 709 thawed oocytes [19], the live birth rate was less than 1%, with a subsequent report announcing the birth of 13 healthy children from 17 pregnancies [90]. Similarly, Tucker et al. [76] also achieved low live-birth rates. A successful regime for oocyte cryopreservation reported 9.2% implantation rate (11 of 120) leading to ongoing pregnancies and subsequent births [24]. Their rates for survival, implantation, and pregnancy were comparable to those in their frozen embryo program, generated from the same cycles. A small vitrification study achieved a 6% live-birth rate (out of 17 oocytes frozen) [54]; another oocytes vitrification program also reported good implantation rates (9.4%; 3 of 32) [70].

D. Results of Cryopreserved Oocytes of Different Maturation Stages

Human oocytes are mostly cryopreserved at metaphase II stage, and the majority of successful pregnancies have been reported from mature oocytes [19,24,54,70]. Meanwhile, the results of human immature oocyte cryopreservation are encouraging [78,79]. The potential of human oocyte cryopreservation at different stages still needs to be explored.

Mature (Metaphase II) Oocytes

Since the first birth was achieved from ICSI-fertilized cryopreserved oocytes [18], fertilization problems related to the freezing were overcome and ICSI has been routinely utilized in fertilizing cryopreserved oocytes [20,21,23,47,61,76,92,93]. Currently, the slow freezing/rapid thawing cryopreservation method with PROH and sucrose, combined with insemination using ICSI, is the preferred method of oocyte cryopreservation.

Early attempts at ultrarapid freezing and vitrification [12,49] were perceived as inferior to slow freezing/rapid thawing. Vitrification of mature oocytes using a cocktail of cryoprotectants produced good survival and fertilization, but no subsequent cleavage [94]. They attributed this to damage to cytoskeletal elements responsible for cell division due to reduction of temperature or cooling combined with the exposure to cryoprotectants. It was only in 1999 that pregnancies resulting from vitrification of mature oocytes using EG and sucrose were reported [53,54], with the latter group reporting the first birth utilizing this technique.

Although parthenogenetic activation of mouse oocytes has been reported after exposure to PROH [95], concerns about human oocytes, especially in PROH protocols [52], may be exaggerated [96]. Tucker et al. [97] justified this observation as a result of delayed fertilization of the oocytes prior to freezing. However, Gook et al. [96] found that PROH can induce parthenogenetic activation, but this activation is not due to PROH alone, and is not elevated in fresh oocytes. This can be caused by temperature variations, or a combined action of both temperature and cryoprotectant [75]. Moreover, in mouse oocytes, PROH can elevate intracellular calcium concentration [98].

Initially, there was concern regarding the increase in polyploidy rates. Al-Hasani et al. [15] reported a high rate of polyploidy using PROH and DMSO as the cryoprotectant (40 and 20%, respectively), but Diedrich et al. [74] observed no increase in polyploidy rates with DMSO. In vitrification using EG, a low polyploidy rate (12%) was observed [53].

Vitrification of human oocytes using EG at different maturational stages showed no clear differences in cryopreservation survival, fertilization, and developmental capacity to achieve pregnancy [53]. Oocytes from both stimulated and unstimulated cycles behaved in a similar fashion after vitrification at various maturational stages, even up to the blastocyst stage [99].

Immature (GV) Oocytes

A higher percentage of surviving cryopreserved oocytes was obtained in mature oocytes compared with intermediately mature or immature oocytes [15], and this coupled with reduced in vitro maturation (IVM) rates makes cryopreservation of immature oocytes seriously inefficient. This was despite the theoretical advantage of freezing the GV oocyte without the cold-sensitive spindle. Furthermore, Park et al. [100] documented increased chromosomal and spindle abnormalities in frozen human GV oocytes. Conversely, others found that immature human oocytes survive freezing and undergo maturation and fertilization with reasonable rates of success [71,78,79,101]. In a later report, Mandelbaum and colleagues [13] found no difference in survival of mature and immature oocytes. However, she reiterated that cryopreservation of immature oocytes will only be beneficial when the outcome from IVM protocols is better controlled. The different survival rates between mature and immature oocytes probably reflect differences in membrane permeability [84].

VI. OVARIAN TISSUE CRYOPRESERVATION AS AN ALTERNATIVE STRATEGY

Ovarian cortical tissue contains large numbers of primordial and primary follicles, which are smaller, lack a zona pellucida and cortical granules, and are less differentiated than mature oocytes. Small oocytes appear to be less sensitive to cryoinjury. Moreover, primordial oocytes have more time to repair the damage in organelles and other structures in the subzero temperatures during their prolonged growth phase after thawing. Human ovarian tissue has been successfully cryopreserved using DMSO, PROH, and EG as cryoprotectants as tested in vitro and in vivo [102,103]. However, the successful method for growing the mature oocytes from the small follicle stage remains a challenge for further research [104–107]. This topic is reviewed in depth elsewhere and is beyond the scope of this chapter.

VII. SAFETY OF OOCYTE CRYOPRESERVATION

Constant debate on the safety of oocyte cryopreservation has revolved around the fact that the fragile microtubules can be depolymerized at low temperatures and on exposure to cryoprotectants, thus damaging the metaphase spindle during cooling [12,40,108]. Despite that fact, high rates of freeze–thaw survival have been reported by Gook et al. [29]. Recently, Porcu [86] claimed that oocyte cryopreservation is becoming a safe and efficient technique; the first few births more than 10 years ago were healthy. Subsequently, Porcu et al. [90] reported obstetric, perinatal outcome and follow-up of children born from cryopreserved oocytes in her center in Italy. Of 17 pregnancies, 11 ended with delivery of 13 healthy children, with normal karyotypes in all but one fetus. There was no major or minor malformation detected. Postnatal growth and physical and intellectual development were normal in all children.

Vitrified oocytes at different maturational stages from both stimulated and unstimulated cycles were capable of reaching the blastocyst stage, and analysis of their chromosomes revealed a normal karyotype [99]. A subsequent paper from the same group reported pregnancy and live births from vitrified oocytes; amniocentesis revealed a normal number of chromosomes with no structural anomalies, and the healthy babies had normal physical profiles [70]. Moreover, fluorescence in situ hybridization (FISH) analysis on embryos from cryopreserved oocytes indicated that the proportion of abnormal embryos after oocyte cryopreservation compared favorably with controls [109]. The application of preimplantation genetic diagnosis (PGD) to embryos derived from cryopreserved oocytes can be an important quality assurance procedure. This may enable selection of euploid embryos, thus increasing implantation rates by discarding those diagnosed as aneuploid. Then recipients of donated cryopreserved oocytes can be provided with greater assurance of a reasonable implantation rate (for details see chapter 7).

REFERENCES

1. Polge C, Smith AU, Parkes AS. Revival of spermatozoa after vitrification and dehydration at low temperatures. Nature (London) 1949; 164: 666.
2. Polge C. Functional survival of fowl spermatozoa after freezing at 79°C. Nature 1951; 167:949–950.
3. Polge C, Lovelock JE. Preservation of bull semen at 79°C. Vet Rec 1952; 64:396–397.
4. Whittingham DG, Leibo SP, Mazur P. Survival of mouse embryos frozen to −196 degrees and −269 degrees C. Science 1972; 178:411–414.
5. Whittingham DG. Fertilization in vitro and development to term of unfertilized mouse oocytes previously stored at −196 degrees C. J Reprod Fertil 1977; 49:89–94.
6. Karlsson JO, Eroglu A, Toth TL, et al. Fertilization and development of mouse oocytes cryopreserved using a theoretically optimized protocol. Hum Reprod 1996; 11:1296–1305.
7. O'Neil L, Paynter SJ, Fuller BJ. Vitrification of mature mouse oocytes: improved results following addition of polyethylene glycol to a dimethyl sulfoxide solution. Cryobiology 1997; 34:295–301.
8. Hotamisligil S, Toner M, Powers RD. Changes in membrane integrity, cytoskeletal structure, and developmental potential of murine oocytes after vitrification in ethylene glycol. Biol Reprod 1996; 55:161–168.
9. Martino A, Songsasen N, Leibo SP. Development into blastocysts of bovine oocytes cryopreserved by ultra-rapid cooling. Biol Reprod 1996; 54:1059–1069.
10. Suzuki T, Boediono A, Takagi M, et al. Fertilization and development of frozen-thawed germinal vesicle bovine oocytes by a one-step dilution method in vitro. Cryobiology 1996; 33:515–524.
11. Trounson A, Mohr L. Human pregnancy following cryopreservation, thawing and transfer of an eight-cell embryo. Nature 1983; 305:707–709.
12. Trounson A. Preservation of human eggs and embryos. Fertil Steril 1986; 46:1–12.

13. Mandelbaum J, Belaisch-Allart J, Junca AM, et al. Cryopreservation in human assisted reproduction is now routine for embryos but remains a research procedure for oocytes. Hum Reprod 1998; 13(suppl 3):161–174.

14. Chen C. Pregnancy after human oocyte cryopreservation. Lancet 1986; 1:884–886.

15. Al-Hasani S, Diedrich K, vander Ven H, et al. Cryopreservation of human oocytes. Hum Reprod 1987; 2:695–700.

16. van Uem JF, Siebzehnrubl ER, Schuh B, et al. Birth after cryopreservation of unfertilized oocytes. Lancet 1987; 1:752–753.

17. Siebzehnruebl ER, Todorow S, van Uem J, et al. Cryopreservation of human and rabbit oocytes and one-cell embryos: a comparison of DMSO and propanediol. Hum Reprod 1989; 4:312–317.

18. Porcu E, Fabbri R, Seracchioli R, et al. Birth of a healthy female after intracytoplasmic sperm injection of cryopreserved human oocytes. Fertil Steril 1997; 68:724–726.

19. Porcu E, Fabbri R, Seracchioli R, et al. Birth of six healthy children after intracytoplasmic sperm injection of cryopreserved human oocytes. Hum Reprod 1998; 13(abstr book 1). 14th Annual Meeting of the ESHRE, Goteburg, June 1998; 124–125.

20. Polak DF, Notrica J, Rubinstein M, et al. Pregnancy after human donor oocyte cryopreservation and thawing in association with intracytoplasmic sperm injection in a patient with ovarian failure. Fertil Steril 1998; 69:555–557.

21. Borini A, Bafaro MG, Bonu MA, et al. Pregnancies after oocytes freezing and thawing. Preliminary Data. Hum Reprod 1998; 13 (abstr book 1). 14th Annual Meeting of the ESHRE, Goteburg, June 1998; 124–125.

22. Antinori S, Dani G, Selman HA, et al. Pregnancies after sperm injection into cryopreserved human human oocytes. Hum Reprod 1998; 13(abstr book 1). 14th Annual Meeting of the ESHRE, Goteburg, June 1998; 157–158.

23. Tucker MJ, Morton PC, Wright G, et al. Clinical application of human egg cryopreservation. Hum Reprod 1998; 13:3156–3159.

24. Yang DS, Blohm PL, Cramer L, et al. A successful human oocyte cryopreservation regime: survival, implantation and pregnancy rates are comparable to that of cryopreserved embryos generated from sibling oocytes. Fertil Steril 1999; 72:(suppl 1, abstr 0-224) S86.

25. Wurfel W, Schleyer M, Krusmann G, et al. [Fertilization of cryopreserved and thawed human oocytes (Cryo-Oo) by injection of spermato-

zoa (ICSI)—medical management of sterility and case report of a twin pregnancy]. Zentralbl Gynakol 1999; 121:444–448.

26. Chia CM, Chan WB, Quah E, et al. Triploid pregnancy after ICSI of frozen testicular spermatozoa into cryopreserved human oocytes: case report. Hum Reprod 2000; 15:1962–1964.

27. Fabbri R, Porcu E, Marsella T, et al. Human oocyte cryopreservation: new perspectives regarding oocyte survival. Hum Reprod 2001; 16: 411–416.

28. Shaw JM, Oranratnachai A, Trouson AO. Cryopreservation of oocytes and embryos. In: Trouson AO, Gardner D, eds., Handbook of In Vitro Fertilization. 2nd ed. Boca Raton: CRC Press, 1999:1–400.

29. Gook DA, Osborn SM, Johnston WI. Cryopreservation of mouse and human oocytes using 1,2-propanediol and the configuration of the meiotic spindle. Hum Reprod 1993; 8:1101–1109.

30. Ruffing NA, Steponkus PL, Pitt RE, et al. Osmometric behavior, hydraulic conductivity, and incidence of intracellular ice formation in bovine oocytes at different developmental stages. Cryobiology 1993; 30: 562–580.

31. Whittingham DG, Siracusa G. The involvement of calcium in the activation of mammalian oocytes. Exp Cell Res 1978; 113:311–317.

32. Whittingham DG. Parthenogenesis in mammals. In: Finn OA, ed., Oxford Reviews of Reproductive Medicine. Oxford, UK: Clarendon Press, 1980:205–231.

33. Dandekar P, Talbot P. Perivitelline space of mammalian oocytes: extracellular matrix of unfertilized oocytes and formation of a cortical granule envelope following fertilization. Mol Reprod Dev 1992; 31:135–143.

34. Vincent C, Pickering SJ, Johnson MH. The hardening effect of dimethylsulphoxide on the mouse zona pellucida requires the presence of an oocyte and is associated with a reduction in the number of cortical granules present. J Reprod Fertil 1990; 89:253–259.

35. Trounson A, Kirby C. Problems in the cryopreservation of unfertilized eggs by slow cooling in dimethyl sulfoxide. Fertil Steril 1989; 52:778–786.

36. Al-Hasani S, Diedrich K. Oocytes storage. In: Grudzinskas JG, Yovich JL, eds. Gametes: The oocyte. Cambridge, UK: Cambridge University Press, 1995.

37. Magistrini M, Szollosi D. Effects of cold and of isopropyl-N-phenylcarbamate on the second meiotic spindle of mouse oocytes. Eur J Cell Biol 1980; 22:699–707.

38. Zenzes MT, Bielecki R, Casper RF, et al. Effects of chilling to 0 degrees C on the morphology of meiotic spindles in human metaphase II oocytes. Fertil Steril 2001; 75:769–777.
39. Van der Elst J, Van den Abeel E, Jacobs R, et al. Effect of 1,2-propanediol and dimethylsulphoxide on the meiotic spindle of the mouse oocyte. Hum Reprod 1988; 3:960–967.
40. Pickering SJ, Braude PR, Johnson MH, et al. Transient cooling to room temperature can cause irreversible disruption of the meiotic spindle in the human oocyte. Fertil Steril 1990; 54:102–108.
41. Kola I, Kirby C, Shaw J, et al. Vitrification of mouse oocytes results in aneuploid zygotes and malformed fetuses. Teratology 1988; 38:467–474.
42. Sathananthan AH, Trounson A, Freemann L, et al. The effects of cooling human oocytes. Hum Reprod 1988; 3:968–977.
43. Saunders KM, Parks JE. Effects of cryopreservation procedures on the cytology and fertilization rate of in vitro-matured bovine oocytes. Biol Reprod 1999; 61:178–187.
44. Bouquet M, Selva J, Auroux M. The incidence of chromosomal abnormalities in frozen-thawed mouse oocytes after in-vitro fertilization. Hum Reprod 1992; 7:76–80.
45. Bouquet M, Selva J, Auroux M. Effects of cooling and equilibration in DMSO, and cryopreservation of mouse oocytes, on the rates of in vitro fertilization, development, and chromosomal abnormalities. Mol Reprod Dev 1995; 40:110–115.
46. Bouquet M, Selva J, Auroux M. Cryopreservation of mouse oocytes: mutagenic effects in the embryo? Biol Reprod 1993; 49:764–769.
47. Porcu E, Fabbri R, Petracchi S, et al. Ongoing pregnancy after intracytoplasmic injection of testicular spermatozoa into cryopreserved human oocytes. Am J Obstet Gynecol 1999; 180:1044–1045.
48. Veeck LL. Freezing of preembryos: early vs late stages. J Assist Reprod Genet 1993; 10:181–185.
49. Pensis M, Loumaye E, Psalti I. Screening of conditions for rapid freezing of human oocytes: preliminary study toward their cryopreservation. Fertil Steril 1989; 52:787–794.
50. Friedler S, Giudice LC, Lamb EJ. Cryopreservation of embryos and ova. Fertil Steril 1988; 49:743–764.
51. Trounson A, Sathananthan H. Human oocyte and embryo freezing. Prog Clin Biol Res 1989; 296:355–366.
52. Imoedemhe DG, Sigue AB. Survival of human oocytes cryopreserved

with or without the cumulus in 1,2-propanediol. J Assist Reprod Genet 1992; 9:323–327.

53. Hong SW, Chung HM, Lim JM, et al. Improved human oocyte development after vitrification: a comparison of thawing methods. Fertil Steril 1999; 72:142–146.

54. Kuleshova L, Gianaroli L, Magli C, et al. Birth following vitrification of a small number of human oocytes: case report. Hum Reprod 1999; 14:3077–3079.

55. Mazur P, Leibo S, Chu EHY. A two-factor hypothesis of freezing injury: evidence from Chinese hamster tissue culture cells. Exp Cell Res 1972; 71:345–355.

56. Wilmut I. The effect of cooling rate, warming rate, cryoprotective agent and stage of development on survival of mouse embryos during freezing and thawing. Life Sci 1972; 11:1071–1079.

57. Trad FS, Toner M, Biggers JD. Effects of cryoprotectants and ice-seeding temperature on intracellular freezing and survival of human oocytes. Hum Reprod 1999; 14:1569–1577.

58. Murayama S, Yamano S, Kobayashi T, et al. Successful freezing of unfertilized mouse oocytes and effect of cocultures in oviducts on development of in vitro fertilized embryos after thawing. J Assist Reprod Genet 1994; 11:156–161.

59. Lim JM, Ko JJ, Hwang WS, et al. Development of in vitro matured bovine oocytes after cryopreservation with different cryoprotectants. Theriogenology 1999; 51:1303–1310.

60. Stachecki JJ, Willadsen SM. Cryopreservation of mouse oocytes using a medium with low sodium content: effect of plunge temperature. Cryobiology 2000; 40:4–12.

61. Gook DA, Schiewe MC, Osborn SM, et al. Intracytoplasmic sperm injection and embryo development of human oocytes cryopreserved using 1,2-propanediol. Hum Reprod 1995; 10:2637–2641.

62. Shaw PW, Fuller BJ, Bernard A, et al. Vitrification of mouse oocytes: improved rates of survival, fertilization, and development to blastocysts. Mol Reprod Dev 1991; 29:373–378.

63. Vajta G, Holm P, Kuwayama M, et al. Open Pulled Straw (OPS) vitrification: a new way to reduce cryoinjuries of bovine ova and embryos. Mol Reprod Dev 1998; 51:53–58.

64. Otoi T, Yamamoto K, Koyama N, et al. Cryopreservation of mature bovine oocytes by vitrification in straws. Cryobiology 1998; 37:77–85.

65. Leibo SP, Martino A, Kobayashi S, et al. Stage-dependent sensitivity of oocytes and embryos to low temperature. Anim.Reprod Sci 1996; 42:45–53.

66. Kasai M, Nishimori M, Zhu SE, et al. Survival of mouse morulae vitrified in an ethylene glycol-based solution after exposure to the solution at various temperatures. Biol Reprod 1992; 47:1134–1139.

67. Shaw PW, Bernard AG, Fuller BJ, et al. Vitrification of mouse oocytes using short cryoprotectant exposure: effects of varying exposure times on survival. Mol Reprod Dev 1992; 33:210–214.

68. Shaw JM, Kuleshova LL, MacFarlane DR, et al. Vitrification properties of solutions of ethylene glycol in saline containing PVP, Ficoll, or dextran. Cryobiology 1997; 35:219–229.

69. Kuleshova LL, MacFarlane DR, Trounson AO, et al. Sugars exert a major influence on the vitrification properties of ethylene glycol-based solutions and have low toxicity to embryos and oocytes. Cryobiology 1999; 38:119–130.

70. Yoon TK, Chung HM, Lim JM, et al. Pregnancy and delivery of healthy infants developed from vitrified oocytes in a stimulated in vitro fertilization-embryo transfer program. Fertil Steril 2000; 74:180–181.

71. Mandelbaum J, Junca AM, Plachot M, et al. Cryopreservation of human embryos and oocytes. Hum Reprod 1988; 3:117–119.

72. Todorow SJ, Siebzehnrubl ER, Spitzer M, et al. Comparative reults on survival of human and animal eggs using different cryoprotectants and freeze-thawing regimens. II. Human. Hum Reprod 1989; 4:812–816.

73. Hunter JE, Bernard A, Fuller B, et al. Fertilization and development of the human oocyte following exposure to cryoprotectants, low temperatures and cryopreservation: a comparison of two techniques. Hum Reprod 1991; 6:1460–1465.

74. Diedrich K, Al-Hasani S, Van der Ven K, et al. Successful in vitro fertilization of frozen-thawed rabbit and human oocytes. In: Feichtinger W, Kemeter P, eds. Future Aspects in Human In Vitro Fertilization. Berlin, Heidelberg: Springer-Verlag, 1987:50–57.

75. Fabbri R, Porcu E, Marsella T, et al. Oocyte cryopreservation. Hum Reprod 1998; 13(suppl 4):4:98–108.

76. Tucker MJ, Wright G, Morton PC, et al. Birth after cryopreservation of immature oocytes with subsequent in vitro maturation. Fertil Steril 1998; 70:578–579.

77. Gook DA, Osborn SM, Bourne H, et al. Fertilization of human oocytes

following cryopreservation; normal karyotypes and absence of stray chromosomes. Hum Reprod 1994; 9:684–691.

78. Toth TL, Lanzendorf SE, Sandow BA, et al. Cryopreservation of human prophase I oocytes collected from unstimulated follicles. Fertil Steril 1994; 61:1077–1082.

79. Toth TL, Baka SG, Veeck LL, et al. Fertilization and in vitro development of cryopreserved human prophase I oocytes. Fertil Steril 1994; 61:891–894.

80. Van der Elst J, Van den Abeel E, Nerinckx S, et al. Parthenogenetic activation pattern and microtubular organization of the mouse oocyte after exposure to 1,2-propanediol. Cryobiology 1992; 29:549–562.

81. Van Blerkom J, Davis PW. Cytogenetic, cellular, and developmental consequences of cryopreservation of immature and mature mouse and human oocytes. Microsc Res Tech 1994; 27:165–193.

82. Candy CJ, Wood MJ, Whittingham DG, et al. Cryopreservation of immature mouse oocytes. Hum Reprod 1994; 9:1738–1742.

83. Frydman N, Selva J, Bergere M, et al. Cryopreserved immature mouse oocytes: a chromosomal and spindle study. Assist Reprod Genet 1997; 14:617–623.

84. Gangrade BK. Oocyte and embryo cryopreservation: Current applications and future outlook. Eds: Diamond MP, DeCherney AH. Infertility and Reproductive Medicine, Clinics of North America. Philadelphia: WB Saunders, 1998; 9:259–273.

85. Ashwood-Smith MJ, Morris GW, Fowler R, et al. Physical factors are involved in the destruction of embryos and oocytes during freezing and thawing procedures. Hum Reprod 1988; 3:795–802.

86. Porcu E. Freezing of oocytes. Curr Opin Obstet Gynecol 1999; 11: 297–300.

87. Young E, Kenny A, Puigdomenech E, et al. Triplet pregnancy after intracytoplasmic sperm injection of cryopreserved oocytes: case report. Fertil Steril 1998; 70:360–361.

88. Chen C. Pregnancies after human oocyte cryopreservation. Ann N Y Acad Sci 1988; 541:541–549.

89. Tucker M, Wright G, Morton P, et al. Preliminary experience with human oocyte cryopreservation using 1,2-propanediol and sucrose. Hum Reprod 1996; 11:1513–1515.

90. Porcu E, Fabbri R, Damiano G, et al. Clinical experience and applications of oocyte cryopreservation. Mol Cell Endocrinol 2000; 169:33–37.

91. Kazem R, Thompson LA, Srikantharajah A, et al. Cryopreservation of human oocytes and fertilization by two techniques: in-vitro fertilization and intracytoplasmic sperm injection. Hum Reprod 1995; 10:2650–2654.

92. Nawroth F, Kissing K. Pregnancy after intracytoplasmatic sperm injection (ICSI) of cryopreserved human oocytes. Acta Obstet Gynecol Scand 1998; 77:462–463.

93. Porcu E, Fabbri R, Ciotti PM, et al. Ongoing pregnancy after intracytoplasmic sperm injection of epididymal spermatozoa into cryopreserved human oocytes. J Assist Reprod Genet 1999; 16:283–285.

94. Hunter JE, Fuller BJ, Bernard A, et al. Vitrification of human oocytes following minimal exposure to cryoprotectants; initial studies on fertilization and embryonic development. Hum Reprod 1995; 10:1184–1188.

95. Shaw JM, Trounson AO. Parthenogenetic activation of unfertilized mouse oocytes by exposure to 1,2-propanediol is influenced by temperature, oocyte age, and cumulus removal. Gamete Res 1989; 24:269–279.

96. Gook DA, Osborn SM, Johnston WI. Parthenogenetic activation of human oocytes following cryopreservation using 1,2-propanediol. Hum Reprod 1995; 10:654–658.

97. Tucker MJ, Morton PC, Sweitzer CL, Wright G. Cryopreservation of human embryos and oocytes. Curr Opin Obstet Gynecol 1995; 7:188–192.

98. Litkouhi B, Winlow W, Gosden RG. Impact of cryoprotective agent exposure on intracellular calcium in mouse oocytes at metaphase II. Cryo-Letters 1999; 20:353–362.

99. Chung HM, Hong SW, Lim JM, et al. In vitro blastocyst formation of human oocytes obtained from unstimulated and stimulated cycles after vitrification at various maturational stages. Fertil Steril 2000; 73:545–551.

100. Park SE, Son WY, Lee SH, et al. Chromosome and spindle configurations of human oocytes matured in vitro after cryopreservation at the germinal vesicle stage. Fertil Steril 1997; 68:920–926.

101. Baka SG, Toth TL, Veeck LL, et al. Evaluation of the spindle apparatus of in-vitro matured human oocytes following cryopreservation. Hum Reprod 1995; 10:1816–1820.

102. Hovatta O, Silye R, Krausz T, et al. Cryopreservation of human ovarian tissue using dimethylsulphoxide and propanediol-sucrose as cryoprotectants. Hum Reprod 1996; 11:1268–1272.

103. Newton H, Aubard Y, Rutherford A, et al. Low temperature storage and grafting of human ovarian tissue. Hum Reprod 1996; 11:1487–1491.
104. Hovatta O, Silye R, Abir R, et al. Extracellular matrix improves survival of both stored and fresh human primordial and primary ovarian follicles in long-term culture. Hum Reprod 1997; 12:1032–1036.
105. Hovatta O, Wright C, Krausz T, et al. Human primordial, primary and secondary ovarian follicles in long-term culture: effect of partial isolation. Hum Reprod 1999; 14:2519–2524.
106. Abir R, Roizman P, Fisch B, et al. Pilot study of isolated early human follicles cultured in collagen gels for 24 hours. Hum Reprod 1999; 14:1299–1301.
107. Gook DA, McCully BA, Edgar DH, et al. Development of antral follicles in human cryopreserved ovarian tissue following xenografting. Hum Reprod 2001; 16:417–422.
108. Johnson MH, Pickering SJ. The effect of dimethylsulphoxide on the microtubular system of the mouse oocyte. Development 1987; 100:313–324.
109. Cobo A, Rubio C, Gerli S, et al. Use of fluorescence in situ hybridization to assess the chromosomal status of embryos obtained from cryopreserved oocytes. Fertil Steril 2001; 75:354–360.
110. Serafini P, Tran C, Tan T, et al. Cryopreservation of human oocytes—A clinical trial. J Assist Reprod Genet 1995; 12(3):PS3-2, 65.
111. Shaw JM, Oranratnachai A, Trounson AO. Fundamental cryobiology of mammalian oocytes and ovarian tissue. Theriogenology 2000; 53:59–72.

9
Treatment of Uterine Anomalies

Carla P. Roberts and John A. Rock
Emory University School of Medicine, Atlanta, Georgia, U.S.A.

I. INTRODUCTION

The müllerian anomalies represent a group of malformations that result
from abnormal formation or incomplete fusion of the müllerian ducts.
Congenital uterine anomalies most commonly are diagnosed after one
or more failed pregnancies, which may manifest as recurrent miscarriage or as mid-trimester loss, or after malpresentation of the fetus at
delivery. Also more frequent are abdominal delivery and postpartum
complications such as retained placenta, subinvolution and hemorrhage. Müllerian malformations lead to gynecologic complaints such
as oligomenorrhea, dysfunctional uterine bleeding, and chronic pelvic
pain and dyspareunia. A surgical emergency may occur, as in the case
of the gestation in a rudimentary uterine horn [1]. Because many, if
not most, women with such malformations have normal reproductive
outcomes, it is important to understand the appropriate techniques used
to diagnose these abnormalities, including septate, bicornuate, didelphic, and unicornuate uteri, and to have a clear clinical perspective
regarding their treatment and subsequent pregnancy rates.

II. NORMAL UTERINE DEVELOPMENT

In the normal embryologic development of the female genital tract,
paramesonephric (müllerian) ducts grow, elongate, and descend from

the lateral aspect of the coelomic cavity toward the midline. The ducts fuse in the midline and then descend to meet the up-growing uterovaginal primordium at the sinovaginal bulb. The sinovaginal bulb elongates to form the vaginal plate, which in turn canalizes to become the vaginal barrel. The fused paramesonephric ducts above the sinovaginal bulb form the uterus. In normal development, the midline fusion of the ducts at the level of the uterus will resorb.

Failure to resorb results in a uterine septum, which also can be associated with a longitudinal vaginal septum if there is failure of resorption caudally. A bicornuate uterus occurs when the müllerian ducts fuse farther caudally than normal. Finally, when there effectively is no fusion of the müllerian ducts, two nonfused hemiuterine cavities result; this anomaly commonly is referred to as uterus didelphys. Obstetricians and gynecologists should consider the possibility of two cervices in any patient with a so-called "double uterus," but the presence of two cervices does not definitively indicate an upper uterine abnormality.

III. CLASSIFICATION

Although numerous classification systems have been suggested for describing uterine anomalies, the most clinically useful system is based chronologically on the embryologic defects occurring in the development of the müllerian ducts. It is best to think of problems with partial development, problems with lateral fusion (obstructive and nonobstructive), and problems with vertical fusion (obstructive and nonobstructive). The American Fertility Society (AFS), in 1988, published the AFS classification that gives a practical, clinical basis for classifying the uterine anomalies and helps define those anomalies that respond best to surgical management [2] (Fig. 1, Table 1).

IV. DIAGNOSIS OF ANOMALIES

The timely and accurate diagnosis of congenital abnormalities primarily depends on the degree to which a physician suspects a problem. Gynecologists often identify patients with uterine anomalies during a

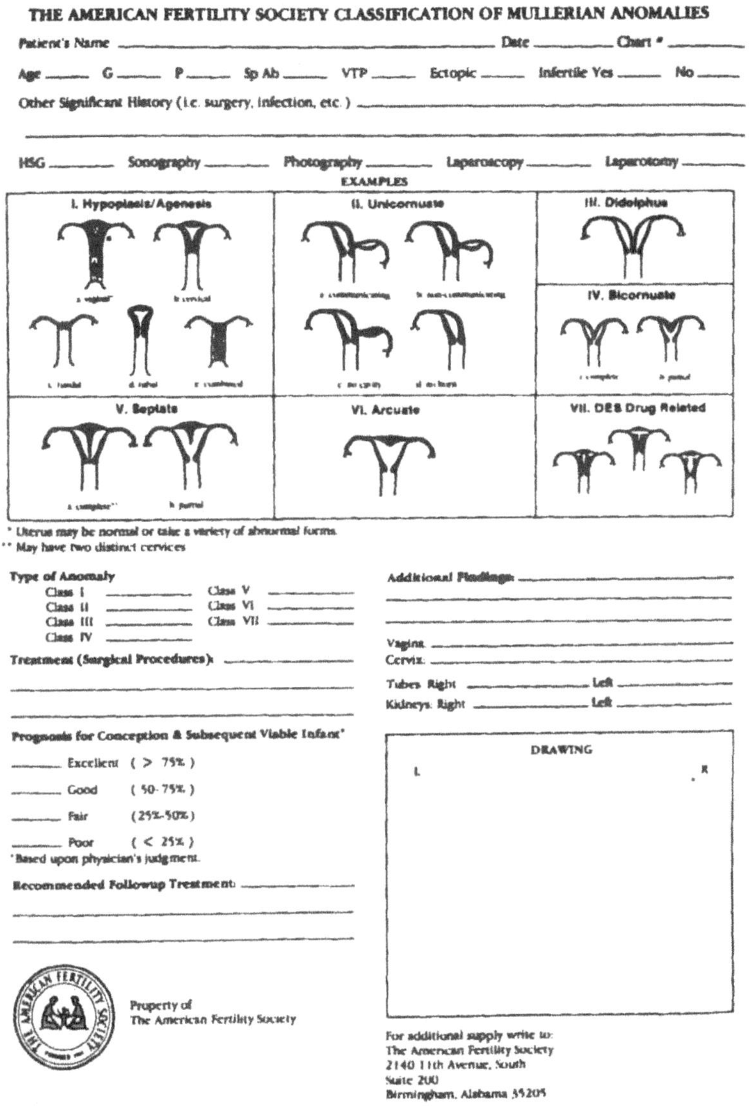

THE AMERICAN FERTILITY SOCIETY CLASSIFICATION OF MULLERIAN ANOMALIES

Patient's Name ______ Date ______ Chart # ______

Age ______ G ______ P ______ Sp Ab ______ VTP ______ Ectopic ______ Infertile Yes ______ No ______

Other Significant History (i.e. surgery, infection, etc.) ______

HSG ______ Sonography ______ Photography ______ Laparoscopy ______ Laparotomy ______

EXAMPLES

I. Hypoplasia/Agenesis

II. Unicornuate

III. Didelphus

IV. Bicornuate

V. Septate

VI. Arcuate

VII. DES Drug Related

* Uterus may be normal or take a variety of abnormal forms.

** May have two distinct cervices

Type of Anomaly

Class I ______ Class V ______

Class II ______ Class VI ______

Class III ______ Class VII ______

Class IV ______

Treatment (Surgical Procedures): ______

Prognosis for Conception & Subsequent Viable Infant*

______ Excellent (> 75%)

______ Good (50-75%)

______ Fair (25%-50%)

______ Poor (< 25%)

*Based upon physician's judgment.

Recommended Followup Treatment: ______

Additional Findings: ______

Vagina: ______

Cervix: ______

Tubes: Right ______ Left ______

Kidneys: Right ______ Left ______

DRAWING

L R

Property of
The American Fertility Society

For additional supply write to:
The American Fertility Society
2140 11th Avenue, South
Suite 200
Birmingham, Alabama 35205

Figure 1 Classification of müllerian anomalies. The physician is able to classify the abnormality by defect, give the treatment for correction and then provide a prognosis for a viable infant. Additional space is provided to describe the entire pelvis and the kidneys. (From Ref. 2.)

Table 1 Classification of Müllerian Anomalies

A. Partial development
    Rokitansky-Kuster Hauser syndrome
    Unicornuate uterus
B. Lateral fusion defects
    Obstructive
        Unilateral vaginal obstruction
        Unilateral vaginal obstruction with a lateral communication
        Unilateral uterine obstruction
    Non-Obstructive
        Uterus didelphys
        Bicornuate uterus
        Septate uterus
        T-shaped uterus
C. Vertical fusion defects
    Obstructive transverse vaginal septum
    Nonobstructive transverse vaginal septum

routine bimanual exam, as in cases of women with a longitudinal vaginal septum; when they present with some manifestation of reproductive failure (recurrent miscarriage or pregnancy associated with a rudimentary uterine horn); or upon discovery of malpresentation of the fetus at delivery. However, women with unexplained preterm labor or fetal loss, or abnormal findings on physical examination of the uterus during pregnancy, often have anomalies that go unsuspected and, as a result, undiagnosed.

V. INCIDENCE

Estimates of the overall incidence of uterine anomalies range from 1 to 5 per 1,000 women. These figures likely underestimate the true incidence, because many women with anomalies do not have reproductive failure and therefore are not diagnosed. For example, when manual exploration of the uterus is performed after a normal delivery, up to 3% of patients may have an anomaly. Anatomic abnormalities of the uterus have been detected in as many as 27% of patients with reproductive failure.

VI. IMPACT ON FERTILITY

The ability to conceive seems to be unimpaired in patients with uterine anomalies, however, there is an increased fetal wastage due to miscarriage. Many times, the primary infertility associated with uterine malformations may be attributed to related disorders such as endometriosis, pelvic adhesions, or ovulatory dysfunction. It is well known that women with outflow tract obstruction, patent tubes, and a functioning endometrium have a high rate of endometriosis [3,4]. Nickerson [5] examined 190 infertile patients and found mild or greater uterine anomalies in 74%. These patients had patent fallopian tubes, normal menses, and no other cause for infertility, and the correlation between an abnormal hysterosalpingogram (HSG) contour and primary infertility was established. Interestingly, the more subtle anomalies have a stronger correlation to infertility than severe fusion defects. Menstrual irregularities and congenital uterine defects have also been associated. After a study of 134 patients with müllerian abnormalities, Sorensen [6] suggested that a congenital defect of steroid receptors in the mildly malformed uterus might yield a syndrome of "steroid unresponsiveness." In addition, diethylstilbestrol (DES)-related anomalies have been associated with oligomenorrhea and primary infertility. Schmidt et al. [7] reviewed the cases of 276 DES-exposed patients and found that 13% demonstrated primary infertility. Impairment in implantation during in vitro fertilization (IVF)–embryo transfer has also been reported in DES-exposed women [8].

VII. IMPACT ON OBSTETRIC FUNCTION

Uterine anomalies are associated with a 15–20% rate of pregnancy wastage. Strassmann [9] noted that reduced intraluminal volume was an important finding in the abnormal uterus and once the limit of expansion of the uterus was reached, abortion resulted. The observation of scant bleeding during resection of a uterine septum is proof of the reduced vascularity of the septum, which may compromise placental perfusion leading to pregnancy loss [10]. This decreased perfusion theory is postulated for the medial surface of a uterine horn as well. Increased uterine irritability and contractibility, possibly associated with alterations in serum cystine aminopeptidase activity, may cause either premature cervical thinning and dilation or placental insufficiency or separation, precipitating spontaneous abortion or premature labor [11].

Lateral fusion defects are the most common identifiable anatomic causes of reproductive failure. It is not known how frequently women with septate or bicornuate uteri actually have reproductive difficulties, because those who do not wish to conceive or who do not have an adverse outcome in pregnancy likely will never be diagnosed. One retrospective review [12] of patients with incidental findings of uterine anomalies during surgery performed for other indications revealed that 93% of patients with didelphic uteri, 84% with bicornuate uteri, and 78% with septate uteri had achieved successful pregnancies. Other studies have suggested a much higher rate of reproductive failure. A review by Musich and Behrman found the corresponding successful pregnancy rates to be only 57% for women with didelphic uteri, 10% for bicornuate uteri, and 15% for septate uteri [13]. The clinical usefulness of this varying data is that many women with uterine anomalies will have a good obstetrical prognosis, but there is a significant risk for further complications in those patients whose uterine malformations are diagnosed because of reproductive failure.

VIII. DIAGNOSIS

Although the physician may suspect a uterine anomaly, history and physical exam are not definitive. The most specific and sensitive test for uterine anomalies is HSG, but the delineation of cavities is limited to the communication of the separate cavities. For example, a noncommunicating horn would not be demonstrated by HSG. In addition, an HSG cannot differentiate between a bicornuate and a septate uterus (Fig. 2). The definitive diagnosis for these anomalies comes from fundal palpation or visualization at the time of surgery.

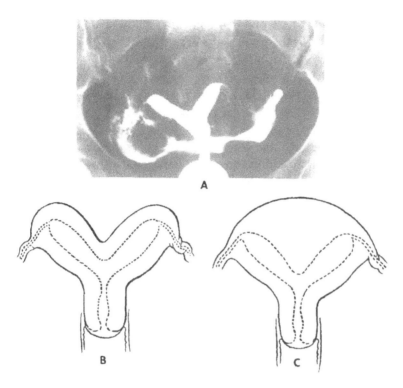

Figure 2 (A) Depiction of a double uterus by hysterosalpingogram. (B) The bicornuate uterus has a heart shaped fundus identifiable by physical exam or laparoscopy. (C) The septate uterus has a broad based fundus identifiable by laparoscopy. (Courtesy of Rock JA. Surgery for anomalies of the müllerian ducts. In: Rock JA, Thompson JD, eds. Telinde's Operative Gynecology, 8th ed. Philadelphia: Lippincott-Raven, 1997:687–729.)

Laparoscopy is helpful in diagnosing the presence or absence of noncommunicating uterine horns and segmental aplastic or hypoplastic anomalies and is essential for documentation of associated pelvic pathology such as pelvic adhesive disease or endometriosis. The value of hysteroscopy in the diagnosis and management of uterine anomalies is most helpful in the resection of uterine septae.

Pelvic ultrasound is helpful in the evaluation of patients with uterine anomalies, particularly in patients who have developed hematocolpos, hematometra, or hematosalpinx. Although there is considerable debate on the issue, some investigators feel that ultrasonography is as reliable as laparoscopy in differentiating a septate from a bicornuate uterus except in the presence of large leiomyomata, marked uterine retroversion, or a large vesicouterorectal fold [14]. In the normal uterus, the linear endometrial stripe progressively widens from the lower uterine segment toward the fundus. With a septate uterus, there usually is a functional separation of the endometrial stripe, with the muscular and connective tissue of the uterus interposed between the two hemiuterine cavities. In the bicornuate uterus, two endometrial stripes without a homogeneous intercavitary portion of the uterus present. In certain cases, the functionally separate horns can be palpated abdominally, but this depends on how thin the patient is and on her ability to tolerate an extensive examination. The thickened endometrial signal in the luteal phase facilitates sonogram interpretation [15]. In addition, ultrasound has been found to be helpful in detecting uterus didelphys and the T-shaped uterus [16].

Urinary tract anomalies occur frequently in association with all types of uterine anomalies except class VII (DES-related) abnormalities. Consequently, intravenous pyelography (IVP) is indicated routinely for patients with suspected müllerian malformations. The reported incidence of renal tract involvement varies from 5% [14] to 100% [17], depending on the anomaly and study. In a review of 42 patients with uterine anomalies, 13 intravenous pyelograms (31%) showed abnormalities, the most common of which was congenital absence of a kidney. Interestingly, class I and II anomalies were associated more frequently with urinary tract malformations than classes III, IV, or V [18].

Magnetic resonance (MR) shows great promise in the workup of uterine anomalies because of its ability optimally to distinguish the shape of the fundal contour as well as to delineate uterine, cervical, and vaginal components. Other anomalies, such as unicornuate uterus and a uterus didelphys with a concealed hemorrhage within noncommunicating horns, müllerian, or cervical agenesis and vaginal septa are also well defined by MR imaging [19–21]. Structures that contain a high concentration of water, as opposed to solid components, tend to have a low to intermediate signal (indicated by a dark color on T1-weighted images) compared to fat, which has a high signal. On T2-weighted images, water-containing tissues tend to be brighter than fat-containing tissues. T1-weighted images provide a general picture of the uterus and other pelvic structures, whereas the specific zones of the uterus (myometrium and endometrium) are best seen with T2-weighted images. Similarly, the endocervix, and thus the entire cervical anatomy, is optimally imaged using T2-weighted sequences. Specific MR patterns have been described for each müllerian anomaly and the urinary system can be visualized concurrently [22]. Although MR imaging may aid in the preoperative workup and discussion between the patient and her surgeon, it is unlikely that imaging studies will replace operative palpation and visualization for the definitive diagnosis.

An HSG is useful in defining the shape and size of the uterine cavity. If two cervices are present, it is recommended to use two tenacula with two separate cannulae to inject radiopaque dye and visualize the separate cavities. If the woman has a single cervix with two cavities demonstrated by other imaging studies, injection of radiopaque contrast will allow the clinician to evaluate for separate and distinct hemiuterine cavities and to determine their communications.

Fluid-contrast ultrasound (sonohysterography) also can be extremely helpful in distinguishing the septate uterus from the bicornuate uterus. This procedure is less expensive, and can be performed in the office at the time of the initial screening examination. The disadvantage is that the fallopian tubes cannot be accurately visualized with fluid-contrast ultrasound.

IX. SPECIFIC ANOMALIES

A. Class I: Agenesis/Dysgenesis

Class I malformations generally result from the abnormal development of the caudal portion of the uterovaginal primordium. The incidence of class I anomalies is estimated to be 1 in 4000–5000. The uterus may be normal or have various abnormal forms. External genitalia and the fallopian tubes are normal. With class Ia malformations, various degrees of agenesis or hypoplasia may cause outflow tract obstruction. The presenting symptom in this class is primary amenorrhea. Approximately 8% of class I anomalies will have a functioning endometrium and present with primary amenorrhea and cyclical pelvic pain (Fig. 3). Hematocolpos, hematometra, hematosalpinx, and endometriosis may develop and manifest as a mass that is palpable on rectal exam. Endometriosis due to outflow tract obstruction may lead to chronic pelvic pain and pelvic adhesive disease. [3].

An imperforate hymen may present as a visible bulging membrane that is often bluish in color as a result of hematocolpos. Pain with an imperforate hymen occurs later than with vaginal agenesis. A diagnosis of a transverse septum must await surgical examination because it resembles a class Ia disorder. Interestingly, a transverse vaginal septum is not associated with an increase in urinary or uterine anomalies. Excision of the transverse septum has been relatively successful

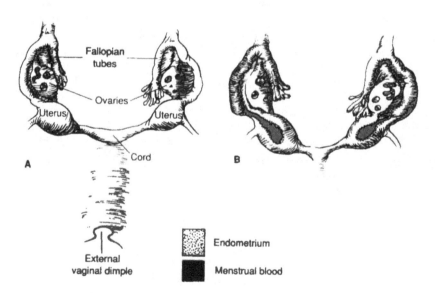

Figure 3 Müllerian agenesis. (A) Bilateral uterine anlagen. (B) Functioning endometrium within the uterine anlagen. (Courtesy of Rock JA. Surgery for anomalies of the müllerian ducts. In: Rock JA, Thompson JD, eds. Telinde's Operative Gynecology, 8th ed. Philadelphia: Lippincott-Raven, 1997:687–729.)

in restoration of menses, pregnancy potential, and vaginal function (Fig. 4).

Pelvic sonography may aid in defining the nature of a pelvic mass secondary to hematocolpos, hematometra, or endometriosis. Laparoscopy is important to determine whether the uterus is normal and to document and treat hematosalpinges and endometriosis. If the uterus or tubes are malformed or diseased to such an extent that reproductive performance will be poor despite neovaginostomy, hysterectomy is the preferred treatment.

A successful vaginal reconstruction depends on the distance from the vaginal pouch and the upper vagina. If the distance is small (as with transverse vaginal septum), incision of the vaginal obstruction with mobilization and anastomosis of the proximal to the distal vaginal is possible. Jeffcoate [23] recommends development of a significant hematocolpos before surgical intervention so that adequate vaginal mucosa will be present for anastomosis. A needle inserted into the hematocolpos may help to identify the appropriate line of entry into the vagina. Care should be taken to make a transverse incision into the vaginal mucosa as far as possible from the urethral meatus. After the surgery, a neoprene dilator should be used daily, in a rotating fashion, along the suture line to avoid strictures and narrowing of the vagina. In cases where the upper and lower vagina are separated by extremely fibrous tissue, neovaginostomy with a split-thickness skin graft should be considered. The classic treatment for vaginal agenesis, in this case, has been the McIndoe vaginoplasty [24]. Successful therapy of any kind is judged by a functional vaginal length of 12 cm or more.

Absence of a cervix (class Ib) in conjunction with a functioning endometrium is extremely rare. A few cases have been reported in patients with a normal vagina (19 cases). Even fewer cases (11 cases) have been reported with cervical agenesis in conjunction with vaginal agenesis. Presenting symptoms are similar to those with obstructive lesions. Attempts to create fistulous tracts from vagina to uterus, to allow for a functioning outflow tract, have had limited success. Farber and Mitchell [25] reported two cases in which they created a fistulous tract, inserting a T tube to maintain patency and allow egress of blood. Zarou et al. [26] using a similar technique, reported a subsequent term pregnancy. Because pregnancies are rare and infection and reoperation

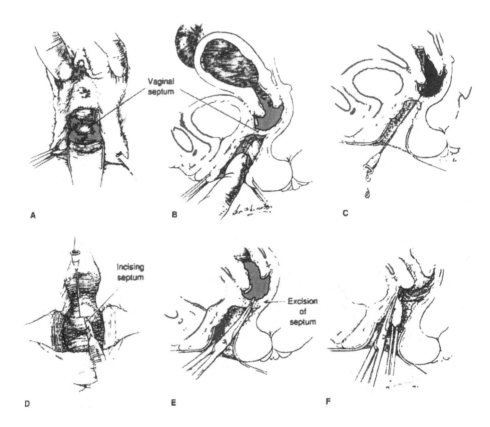

A   B   C

D   E   F

Vaginal
septum

Incising
septum

Excision
of
septum

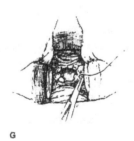

G

are common, hysterectomy is the optimal long-term therapy. With the advances of assisted reproductive technique (ART), if pregnancy is desired, gamete intrafallopian transfer should be considered if the uterus and tubes appear normal.

Few cases of fundal agenesis (class Ic) have been reported, possibly because there is no treatment available and usually no indication for surgery. The obvious symptoms of class Ic anomalies are amenorrhea and sterility. A hypoplastic cervix without an os and a palpably small fundus may be found on examination.

Congenital tubal agenesis (class Id) is rare. Isolated bilateral tubal agenesis has never been reported. Unilateral tubal agenesis has been reported with a unicornuate uterus without a contralateral horn, however congenital unilateral tubal agenesis with a normal uterus and bilaterally normal ovaries has not been reported. Autoamputation of the fallopian tube secondary to adjacent ovarian torsion and infarction can occur. In these cases, a small section of calcified ovary may be found in the cul-de-sac. Segmental tubal agenesis has been observed and these patients are assumed to have one normal tube unless it is known to have been damaged. If so, anastomosis may be indicated in the tube with segmental agenesis, but such a tube carries an increased risk of ectopic pregnancy and should be removed or repaired at the reproductive surgeon's discretion.

Combined müllerian agenesis or hypoplasia (class Ie) consists of vaginal agenesis associated with a rudimentary uterus. Fallopian tubes generally are present and appear normal. This anomaly has been termed the Mayer-Rokitansky-Küster-Hauser (MRKH) syndrome. Although

---

Figure 4 Repair of a transverse vaginal septum. (A) The neovaginal space is examined revealing a transverse vaginal septum. (B) Palpation of the septum. (C) A needle is inserted into the bulging hematocolpos. (D) A knife is used to enter the vaginal mucosa. (E and F) The septum is excised by sequential clamping and cutting. It is then removed. (G) The excised areas are sutured with interrupted sutures of 2-0 vicryl. (Courtesy of Rock JA. Surgery for anomalies of the müllerian ducts. In: Rock JA, Thompson JD, eds. Telinde's Operative Gynecology, 8th ed. Philadelphia: Lippincott-Raven, 1997:687–729.)

vaginal agenesis may occur in combination with a functioning uterus (class Ia), the combined absence is more common, representing 80%–90% of reported cases relating to vaginal agenesis. Primary amenorrhea and sterility are the usual presenting symptoms, although in unusual circumstances a rudimentary structure containing functioning endometrium will cause cyclic pelvic pain. External genitalia are normal. The vagina ends in a blind pouch, typically with a depth of 1 to 2 cm. Rectal or rectovaginal examination may sometimes reveal a 2- to 3-cm nodular structure in the cul-de-sac representing the undeveloped anlage of the uterus. A palpable pelvic mass may represent a pelvic kidney because major urinary tract anomalies occur with a frequency of approximately 15%. If minor urinary tract anomalies are included, the frequency increases to about 40%. Sonography or MR imaging may be helpful in determining the presence of a uterus.

The MRKH syndrome is associated with shortness of stature, severe bony abnormalities involving the spine, and sometimes deafness [27]. The karyotype is typically normal 46 XX. The appearance of the syndrome suggests that arrest of development occurs at about 7 weeks of fetal age (9 weeks after the last menstrual period).

These patients have no reproductive potential without the help of ART, although functional improvement of the vagina can be achieved as with class Ia anomalies. The surgical treatment of choice is the McIndoe vaginoplasty [24]. Recently, Roberts et al. reviewed 51 cases of patients with müllerian agenesis and demonstrated a 91.9% success rate with the Ingram method of vaginal dilation [28] (Fig. 5). Other methods of dilation and surgical repair have been attempted but yield lower degrees of success. A laparoscopy is necessary only to evaluate cyclic pelvic pain. Removal of uterine anlagen containing functional endometrium is generally the only indicated surgical procedure.

B. Class II: Unicornuate

Class II anomalies result from normal differentiation of only one müllerian duct. The other develops either partially (class IIa, IIb, or IIc) or not at all (class IId). The rudimentary horn has no cavity. Symptoms vary depending on the degree of obstruction to menstrual outflow. Patients with a noncommunicating functional horn (class IIb) are at risk

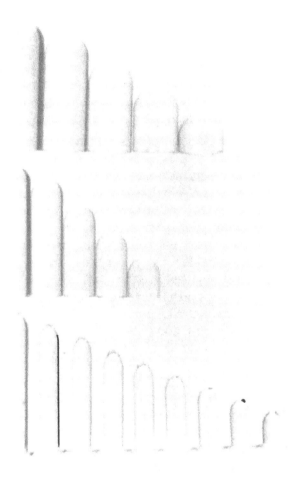

Figure 5 A set of Ingram vaginal dilators. The set includes 19 dilators of varying lengths and widths. (Courtesy of Rock JA. Surgery for anomalies of the müllerian ducts. In: Rock JA, Thompson JD, eds. Telinde's Operative Gynecology, 8th ed. Philadelphia: Lippincott-Raven, 1997:687–729.)

for the development of hematometra, hematosalpinx, endometriosis, and rudimentary horn pregnancies.

Many investigators have assumed that the incidence of spontaneous abortion would be the same for unicornuate and didelphic uteri, and therefore they combine data for these two groups under the heading hemiuterus. A recent report comparing 29 women with unicornuate uteri and 25 women with didelphic uteri is consistent with that assumption [29]. Reported abortion rates range from 26 to 34%, with a total of 119 pregnancies in 50 patients and an overall abortion rate of 33% [14]. In studies that report only on unicornuate uteri, the abortion rate ranges from 8 to 86% [30]. In 31 patients with 60 pregnancies there was an overall fetal loss rate of 48%. It is not possible to determine from available data whether the incidence of abortion was higher in the first than in the second trimester. A high rate in the second trimester might indicate the existence of an incompetent cervix. Whether the presence of a rudimentary horn predisposes to pregnancy wastage is unclear. The reproductive performance may be routinely poor whether or not there is a rudimentary horn [18]. The presence of a rudimentary horn with functioning endometrium increases the risk of morbidity secondary to either endometriosis or a pregnancy in the rudimentary horn. In a review of the world literature, O'Leary and O'Leary [31] found reports of 327 rudimentary horn gestations, noting that 89% of the abnormal uteri had ruptured by the end of the second trimester and that only 1% of the pregnancies resulted in live, term births. They estimated that 90% of rudimentary horns in unicornuate uteri are noncommunicating. Premature labor has long been associated with a unicornuate uterus, with reported rates ranging from 8 to 38%. Abnormal presentation (usually breech) may occur in up to 67% of cases. The reported live birth rate ranges from 14 to 100%. Combined data from 11 reports yield a live birth rate of 54% [29,32–41].

Physical exam reveals normal external genitalia, vagina, and cervix. In those patients having a rudimentary horn, the unicornuate uterus will be found to deviate to the right or the left and generally will be smaller than a normal uterus. A small, hard pelvic mass (the rudimentary horn) may be felt in the contralateral adnexa. A pelvic mass may represent a hematometra, hematosalpinx, or a pelvic kidney. The final diagnosis will depend upon HSG and laparoscopy. Sonography may be helpful, particularly to detect a noncommunicating functional horn.

No therapy is universally advocated for the treatment of preterm delivery, but cervical cerclage has been suggested for those patients with a history consistent with an incompetent cervix. Removal of a communicating or nonfunctional rudimentary horn is not indicated initially in the infertile patient because most patients conceive without difficulty. If, however the patient is infertile and no other contributing factors can be identified, reconstructive surgery may be offered, although its benefits are poorly substantiated. This procedure is indicated for all patients, infertile or otherwise, with a noncommunicating functional horn to prevent the development of hematometra, hematosalpinx, and endometriosis.

C. Class III: Didelphys

Complete failure of the müllerian ducts to fuse in the midline gives rise to a uterus didelphys with normal differentiation of both ducts, resulting in duplication of the uterus and cervix. In about 75% of cases of uterus didelphys, the vagina is septate as well.

Dyspareunia may be associated with a vaginal septum; although patients with this anomaly generally are asymptomatic, a patient may occasionally present with lower abdominal pain or dysmenorrhea and a bulging mass at the vaginal outlet (hematocolpos). It is interesting that the diagnosis of unilateral vaginal obstruction (complete or incomplete) is rarely considered by the initial treating physician. One study of 11 patients revealed that the age of presenting symptoms was 15.5 years; however, the age of definitive diagnosis and treatment was 23.7 years [42]. These patients may also demonstrate unilateral hematocolpos and rarely, hematometra, hematosalpinx, and endometriosis. With incomplete obstruction, a foul, mucopurulent discharge may occur intermittently. Less than 100 such cases have been reported in the literature. Most of the cases were associated with a didelphic uterus, although some cases have been associated with bicornuate or septate uteri.

The reproductive outcomes are similar in unicornuate and didelphic uteri. Combined data from reported series suggest a 35% spontaneous abortion rate, a 19% rate of preterm delivery, and a live birth rate of 60% [30,32].

The presence of a vaginal septum suggests a didelphic uterus but is not diagnostic because it may occur alone or in conjunction with a complete septate or bicornuate uterus. Similarly, the presence of two cervices implies uterus didelphys, but such malformations can also occur with septate or bicornuate uteri. Pelvic exam and sonography may be helpful in interpreting the HSG, but laparoscopy (or MR imaging) may be necessary for definitive diagnosis.

Rock and Jones [43] reported congenital absence of a kidney in 9% of their patients with double uteri for whom IVP was obtained. They concluded that ipsilateral renal agenesis is observed almost without exception when a longitudinal vaginal septum causes complete or almost complete unilateral vaginal obstruction [44].

Because there is a live birth rate of 60%, surgical therapy is rarely performed. For those patients who demonstrate multiple fetal wastage, some recommend a modified Strassmann procedure or cervical cerclage. In some cases, a vaginal septum interferes with proper assessment of the patient with a uterine anomaly. HSG may be difficult or impossible. For this reason, incision of the septum may be performed at the time of laparoscopy. Excision of the asymptomatic septum is usually not necessary.

D. Class IV: Bicornuate

When two normally differentiated ducts partially fuse in the region of the fundus, the result is a bicornuate uterus. The division may be complete to the cervix (class IVa) or a partial (class IVb). The true incidence of bicornuate uterus is difficult to assess because information about the bicornuate uterus and the septate uterus are usually combined under the designation of double uterus. In the past, bicornuate uteri were thought to be relatively common, but more recent experience with HSG and laparoscopy indicates that many anomalies once considered bicornuate are really septate.

Normally, the only symptoms are obstetric problems unless a symptomatic vaginal septum is present. Ability to conceive is not impaired. Data from studies reporting on double uteri (including both bicornuate and septate) indicate a 61% abortion rate in 1914 pregnancies. When a bicornuate uterus was definitively diagnosed by laparoscopy, 35% of 313 pregnancies aborted, suggesting a higher abortion rate associated with septate than bicornuate uteri [30]. Comparing incomplete and complete bicornuate uteri, Acién [32] found a higher abortion rate in incomplete bicornuate uteri. In addition, with uteri specifically diagnosed as bicornuate, 23% of 203 pregnancies that were neither aborted nor ectopic were delivered prematurely [30]. Malpresentation occurs in about 20% of pregnancies.

Palpation of two distinct horns on bimanual examination or visualization of two distinct horns at laparoscopy is usually diagnostic. HSG and sonography usually do not differentiate between bicornuate and septate uteri. The frequency of IVP abnormalities in these patients is approximately 20%.

The recommended therapy for class IV abnormalities is the Strassmann procedure. This procedure has the advantage of not requiring excision of uterine tissue and thus not reducing the potential uterine space (Fig. 6). Strassmann [9] reported his experience with uterine unification procedures, noting an increase in the live birth rate from 2% to 82% postoperatively. The effectiveness of cervical cerclage in this group of patients has not been established.

E. Class V: Septate

The septate uterus is divided by a longitudinal septum, either partially (class Vb) or completely (class Va, septum to internal os with possibly two distinct cervices). The most imposing feature of class V anomalies is the rate of spontaneous abortion, which is reported to be in excess of 60% [30]. The high abortion rate may be associated with decreased functional uterine volume or with inadequate blood supply to the relatively avascular septum [30]. Inability to conceive is an uncommon complaint in the absence of endometriosis, pelvic adhesive disease, or leiomyomata. Septate uteri are associated with other obstetric complications, including preterm labor, malpresentation and retained placenta.

A broad uterine fundus felt on bimanual exam may suggest a septate uterus, but HSG and laparoscopy (or MR imaging) are usually required to distinguish between a septate and a bicornuate uterus. Occa-

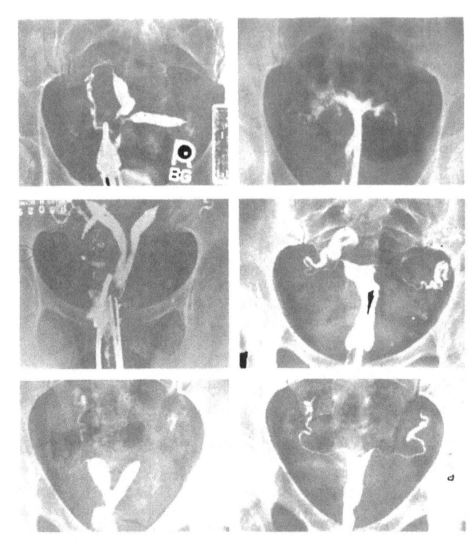

Figure 6   Hysterosalpingogram of three different bicornuate uterine cavities before and after reunification. (Courtesy of Rock JA. Surgery for anomalies of the müllerian ducts. In: Rock JA, Thompson, JD, eds. Telinde's Operative Gynecology, 8th ed. Philadelphia: Lippincott-Raven, 1997:687–729.)

sionally, a vaginal septum is found. The incidence of associated renal anomalies is probably about 20% [30].

In the past, the recommended therapy was the Jones metroplasty [45] or the Tomkins procedure [46]. More recently, hysteroscopic resection of the uterine septum has become the treatment of choice [47] (Fig. 7). Rock et al. reviewed 21 patients with a history of repeated pregnancy losses and a class Va septum who underwent hysteroscopic uter-

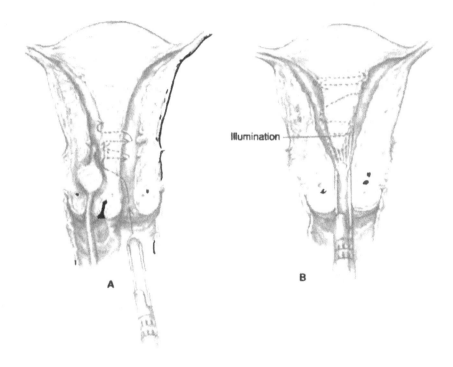

Figure 7 Hysteroscopic resection of a uterine septum. (A) A foley catheter is placed inside one cavity of a complete septate uterus (class Va). The resectoscope is entered into the other cavity and the septum is incised until the foley catheter is seen in the opposite cavity. The septum is excised until both tubal ostia are visualized. (B) A partial septum (class Vb) can be easily excised by the resectoscope. (Courtesy of Rock JA. Surgery for anomalies of the müllerian ducts. In: Rock JA, Thompson JD, eds. Telinde's Operative Gynecology, 8th ed. Philadelphia: Lippincott-Raven, 1997:687–729.)

ine septum resection. Fourteen of the fifteen women attempting pregnancy delivered viable infants and the fifteenth patient had an ongoing pregnancy at the time of publication [48].

F. Class VI: Arcuate

The class VI anomalies consist of minimal uterine structural changes with no external dimpling and minimal changes in uterine cavity shape. There is little evidence implicating the arcuate uterus as a cause of reproductive failure, although one report suggests a significant rate of spontaneous abortion [32]. The AFS classification includes this malformation in its categories and it is reported in those cases in which its presence was believed to be clinically significant.

G. Class VII: DES Related

After the synthesis of DES in 1938, clinical studies suggested a beneficial effect in the treatment of threatened abortions, prevention of spontaneous abortion in patients with a history of repeated pregnancy loss [49], and a reduction of late pregnancy complications such as toxemia, preterm delivery, postmaturity, and stillbirth [50]. Subsequent controlled studies failed to confirm such benefits and, in fact, documented an association of DES with adverse obstetrical outcomes [51,52].

In 1970, the occurrence of clear cell adenocarcinoma of the vagina in seven girls aged 14–22 years was reported [53], which exceeded the total number of all such cancers previously reported in this age range [54]. Between 1970 and 1980, numerous descriptions of anatomic and functional abnormalities of both the lower and the upper müllerian tracts of women exposed to DES in utero appeared.

Specific changes in the contour of the uterine cavity have been reported, and abnormal HSG findings are likely to be present if gross anatomic cervical or vaginal epithelial changes have occurred [55]. Asymmetric myometrial hypertrophy appears to be responsible for abnormalities in the contour of the uterine cavity [56]. Compared with controls, women exposed to DES in utero have higher rates of ectopic pregnancy, spontaneous abortion, preterm delivery, and perinatal death, although more than 80% of exposed women who conceive eventually carry a pregnancy that results in a live-born infant [54]. Those patients with an abnormal uterine contour are at a higher risk for adverse outcome than exposed women with a normal pelvic radiograph. An elevated second trimester abortion rate is suggestive but not diagnostic of cervical incompetence [57,58]. DES exposure in utero has not been associated with abnormalities of the urinary tract.

Menstrual abnormalities, predominantly oligomenorrhea, reportedly occur more frequently in DES-exposed women. It has been suggested that effects of DES on the developing hypothalamic–pituitary axis may result in disturbed gonadotropin cyclicity [59]. Other investigators have reported an increased incidence of dysmenorrhea that may be related to a constricted outflow tract [60].

Primary infertility may be increased among DES-exposed women. Bibbo et al. [59] reported nonexposed women have a higher live pregnancy rate than DES-exposed women (33 versus 18%), although there was no difference in reported problems with conceiving between the two groups. Herbst et al. [61] reported a higher rate of primary infertility among DES-exposed women (16%) compared with controls (6%), although no causative factor has been identified. Impaired implantation has been suggested by Karande et al. [62], who found lower implantation rates in DES-exposed women treated with IVF than in nonexposed women undergoing IVF during the same time period. In addition, a worse prognosis was associated with HSG findings of uterine constrictions and the combination of a T shape and constriction.

Experience with surgical correction of DES-associated uterine abnormalities is limited, and surgery is generally discouraged. A history consistent with cervical incompetence may be an indication for cervical cerclage, but prophylactic cerclage placement is unwarranted. Jones [63] recommends metroplasty for patients with a T-shaped uterus who have not achieved a successful pregnancy. Using a slight modification of the Strassmann procedure, the center part of the crossbar of the T is unroofed and the uterus is reunited in the midline creating a symmetrical I-shaped cavity (Fig. 8). A recent report described hysteroscopic lateral metroplasty in eight patients with uterine changes associated

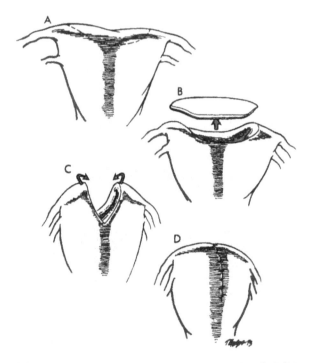

Figure 8 Technique for the surgical repair of a DES-exposed uterine cavity. (Courtesy of Rock JA. Surgery for anomalies of the müllerian ducts. In: Rock JA, Thompson JD, eds. Telinde's Operative Gynecology, 8th ed. Philadelphia: Lippincott-Raven, 1997:687–729.)

with DES exposure, although that history could be confirmed in only five of the patients [64]. Preliminary follow-up indicates a significant improvement in pregnancy outcome.

X. SUMMARY

The reproductive implications of congenital anomalies of the uterus are profound. Accurate diagnosis is critical, and aggressive treatment often will produce excellent results for those women with prior reproductive failure.

The approach to patients who have incidental diagnoses without previous failure depends on the configuration of the uterus and the patient's preferences. In the absence of previous reproductive failure, patients with a bicornuate uterus do not need surgical correction. Conversely, it is reasonable to perform a hysteroscopic metroplasty on patients with a septate uterus even without prior reproductive failure, because the pregnancy loss rates are much higher.

The use of imaging techniques and a working relationship with a knowledgeable group of radiologists is helpful when caring for these patients. Gynecologists should consult with experienced colleagues prior to any surgical procedure when the diagnosis is unclear.

REFERENCES

1. Johansen K. Pregnancy in a rudimentary horn" two case reports. Obstet Gynecol 1969; 34:805–808.
2. American Fertility Society. The American Fertility Society classifications of adnexal adhesions, distal tubal occlusion, tubal occlusion secondary to tubal ligation, tubal pregnancies, mullerian anomalies and intrauterine adhesions. Fertil Steril 1988; 49:944.
3. Olive DL, Henderson DY. Endometriosis and müllerian anomalies. Obstet Gynecol 1987; 69:412–415.
4. Fedele L, Bianchi S, DiNola G, Franchi D. Candiani GB. Endometriosis and nonobstructive müllerian anomalies. Obstet Gynecol 1992; 79:515–517.
5. Nickerson CW. Infertility and uterine contour. Am J Obstet Gynecol 1977; 129:268–273.
6. Sorensen SS. Minor müllerian anomalies and oligomenorrhea in infertile women: a new syndrome. Am J Obstet Gynecol 1981; 140:636–644.
7. Schmidt G, Fowler WC, Talbert LM, Edelman DA. Reproductive history of women exposed to diethylstilbestrol in utero. Fertil Steril 1980; 33: 21–24.
8. Karande VC, Lester RG, Muasher SJ, Jones DL, Acosta AA, Jones HW Jr. Are implantation and pregnancy outcome impaired in diethylstilbestrol-exposed women after in vitro fertilization and embryo transfer? Fertil Steril 1990; 54:287–291.
9. Strassmann EO. Fertility and unification of double uterus. Fertil Steril 1966; 17:165–176.

10. Hunt JE, Wallach EE. Uterine factors in infertility—an overview. Clin
    Obstet Gynecol 1974; 17:44–64.
11. Blum M. Comparative study of serum CAP activity in pregnancy in
    malformed and normal uterus. J Perinat Med 1978; 6:165–168.
12. Thompson JP, Smith RA, Welch JS. Reproductive ability after metro-
    plasty. Obstet Gynecol 1966; 28:363–368.
13. Musich JR, Behrman SJ. Obstetric outcome before and after metroplasty
    in women with uterine anomalies. Obstet Gynecol 1978; 52:63–66.
14. Fedele L, Ferrazzi E, Dorta M. Ultrasonography in the differential diag-
    nosis of "double" uteri. Fertil Steril 1988; 50:361–364.
15. Reuter KL, Daly DC, Cohen SM. Septate versus bicornuate uteri: errors
    in imaging diagnosis. Radiology 1989; 172:749–752.
16. Shapiro BS, DeCherney AH. Ultrasound and infertility. J Reprod Med
    1989; 34:151–155.
17. Woolf RB, Allen WM. Concomitant malformations. The frequent, si-
    multaneous occurrence of congenital malformations of the reproductive
    and urinary tracts. Obstet Gynecol 1953; 2:236–239.
18. Buttram VC, Gibbons WE. Mullerian anomalies: a proposed classifica-
    tion (an analysis of 144 cases). Fertil Steril 1979; 32:40–46
19. Mintz MC, Thickman DI, Gussman D. MR evaluation of uterine anoma-
    lies. Am J Roent 1987:148:287–290.
20. Fedele L, Dorta M, Brioschi D. Magnetic resonance evaluation of double
    uteri. Obstet Gynecol 1989; 74: 844–847.
21. Carrington BM, Hricak H, Nuruddin RN. Mullerian duct anomalies:
    MRI imaging evaluation. Radiology 1990; 176:715–720.
22. Doyle MB. Magnetic resonance imaging in müllerian fusion defects. J
    Reprod Med 1992; 37:33–38
23. Jeffcoate TN. Advancement of the upper vagina in the treatment of hem-
    atocolpos and hematometra caused by vaginal aplasia. Pregnancy fol-
    lowing the construction of an artificial vagina. J Obstet Gynaecol Br
    Commonw 1969; 76:961–968.
24. McIndoe AH. The treatment of congenital absence and obliterative con-
    ditions of the vagina. Br J Plast Surg 1949; 2:254–259.
25. Farber M, Mitchell GW. Anomalies of the kidney and the ureters. Clin
    Obstet Gynecol 1978; 21:831–843.
26. Zarou GS, Esposito JM, Zarou DM. Pregnancy following the surgical
    correction of congenital atresia of the cervix. Int J Gynecol Obstet 1973;
    11:143–146.
27. Park IJ, Jones HW, Nager GT, Chen SC, Hussels IE. A new syndrome
    in two unrelated females: Klippel-Feil deformity, conductive deafness

and absent vagina. In Birth Defects: Original Articles VIII. New York: Alan R. Liss, Inc, 1971:311.

28. Roberts CP, Haber M, Rock JA. Vaginal creation for müllerian agenesis. Am J Obstet Gynecol 2001; 185(6):1349–1353.

29. Moutos DM, Damewood MD, Schlaff WD, Rock JA. A comparison of the reproductive outcome between women with a unicornuate uterus and women with a didelphic uterus. Fertil Steril 1992; 58:88–93.

30. Buttram VC Jr, Reiter RC. Uterine anomalies. In: Surgical Treatment of the Infertile Female. Baltimore: Williams and Wilkins, 1985:149–199.

31. O'Leary JL, O'Leary JA. Rudimentary horn pregnancy. Obstet Gynecol 1963; 22:371–374.

32. Acién P. Reproductive performance of women with uterine malformations. Hum Reprod 1993; 8:122–126.

33. Heinonen PK, Saarikoski S, Pystynen P. Reproductive performance of women with uterine anomalies. Acta Obstet Gynecol Scand 1982; 61:157–162.

34. Fedele L, Zamberletti D, Vercellini P, Dorta M, Candiani GB. Reproductive performance of women of women with unicornuate uterus. Fertil Steril 1987; 47:416–419.

35. Andrews MC, Jones HW Jr. Impaired reproductive performance of the unicornuate uterus: intrauterine growth retardation, infertility and recurrent abortion in five cases. Am J Obstet Gynecol 1982; 144:173–175.

36. Beernink FJ, Beernink HE, Chinn A. Uterus unicornis with uterus solidaris. Obstet Gynecol 1976; 47:651–653.

37. Buttram VC Jr. Mullerian anomalies and their management. Fertil Steril 1983; 40:159–163.

38. Stein AL, March CM. Pregnancy outcome in women with müllerian duct anomalies. J Reprod Med 1990; 35:411–414.

39. Ludmir J, Samuel P, Brooks S, Mennuti MT. Pregnancy outcome of patients with uncorrected uterine anomalies managed in a high-risk obstetric setting. Obstet Gynecol 1990; 75:910–916.

40. Musich JR, Behrman SJ. Obstetric outcome before and after metroplasty in women with uterine anomalies. Obstet Gynecol 1978; 52:63–66.

41. Maneschi M, Maneschi F, Fuca G. Reproductive impairment of women with unicornuate uterus. Acta Eur Fertil 1988; 19:273–275.

42. Toaff R. A major genital malformation: Communicating uteri. Obstet Gynecol 1988; 43:167.

43. Rock JA, Jones HW. The clinical management of the double uterus. Fertil Steril 1977; 28:798–806.

44. Rock JA, Jones HW. The double uterus associated with an obstructed hemivagina and ipsilateral renal agenesis. Am J Obstet Gynecol 1980; 138:339–342.

45. Jones HW Jr, Jones GES. Double uterus as an etiological factor of repeated abortion, indication for surgical repair. Am J Obstet Gynecol 1956; 72:865.

46. Tomkins P. Comments on the bicornuate uterus and twinning. Surg Clin North Am 1962; 42:1049–1052.

47. March CM. Hysteroscopy. J Reprod Med 1992; 3:293–312.

48. Rock JA, Roberts CP, Hesla JS. Hysteroscopic metroplasty of the class Va uterus with preservation of the cervical septum. Fertil Steril 1999; 72:942–945.

49. Smith OW. Diethylstilbestrol in the prevention and treatment of complications of pregnancy. Am J Obstet Gynecol 1948; 56:821–824.

50. Smith OW, Smith G, Van S. The influence of diethylstilbestrol on the progress and outcome of pregnancy based on a comparison of treated with untreated primigravidas. Am J Obstet Gynecol 1949; 58:994–998.

51. Dieckmann WJ, Davis ME, Rynkiewicz LM. Does the administration of diethylstilbestrol during pregnancy have the therapeutic value? Am J Obstet Gynecol 1953; 66:1062–1065.

52. Brackbold Y, Berendes HW. Dangers of diethylstilbestrol: review of a 1953 paper. Lancet 1978; 2:520–524.

53. Herbst AL, Scully RE. Adenocarcinoma of the vagina in adolescence: a report of seven cases including six clear cell carcinomas (so-called mesonephromas). Cancer 1970; 25:745–757.

54. Stillman RJ. In utero exposure to diethylstilbestrol: adverse effects on the reproductive tract and reproductive performance in male and female offspring. Am J Obstet Gynecol 1982; 142:905–921.

55. Kaufman RH, Binder GL, Gray PM Jr, Adam E. Upper genital tract changes associated with exposure in utero to diethylstilbestrol. Am J Obstet Gynecol 1977; 128:51–59.

56. Kaufman RH, Adam E, Binder BL, Gerthoffer E. Upper genital tract changes and pregnancy outcome in offspring exposed in utero to diethylstilbestrol. Am J Obstet Gynecol 1980; 137:299–308.

57. Stein AL, March CM. Pregnancy outcome in women with müllerian duct anomalies. J Reprod Med 1990; 35:411–414.

58. Herbst AL, Hubby MM, Blough RR, Azizi F. A comparison of pregnancy experience in DES-exposed and DES-unexposed daughters. J Reprod Med 1980; 24:62–69.

59. Bibbo M, Gill WB, Azizi F, Blough R, Fang VS, Rosenfield RL, Schumacher GF, Sleeper K, Sonek MG, Wied GL. Follow-up study of male and female offspring of DES-exposed mothers. Obstet Gynecol 1977; 49:1–8.

60. Haney AF, Hammond CB, Soules MR, Creasman WT. Diethylstilbestrol-induced upper genital tract abnormalities. Fertil Steril 1979; 31: 142–146.

61. Herbst AL, Hubby MM, Azizi F, Makii MM. Reproductive and gynecologic surgical experience in diethylstilbestrol-exposed daughters. Am J Obstet Gynecol 1981; 141:1019–1028.

62. Karande VC, Lester RG, Muasher SJ, Jones DL, Acosta AA, Jones HW Jr. Are implantation and pregnancy outcome in diethylstilbestrol-exposed women after in vitro fertilization and embryo transfer? Fertil Steril 1990; 54:287–291.

63. Jones HW Jr. Reconstruction of congenital uterovaginal anomalies. In Rock JA, Murphy AA, Jones HW Jr, eds. Female Reproductive Surgery. Baltimore: Williams and Wilkins, 1992:246–258.

64. Nagel TC, Malo JW. Hysteroscopic metroplasty in the diethylstilbestrol-exposed uterus and similar nonfusion anomalies: Effects on subsequent reproductive performance; a preliminary report. Fertil Steril 1993; 59: 502–506.

10
Practical Management of Ectopic Pregnancy

Mazen Bisharah
*McGill University and McGill University Health Centre,
Montreal, Quebec, Canada*

Togas Tulandi
McGill University, Montreal, Quebec, Canada

Ectopic pregnancy (EP) is a major health problem for women of reproductive age and is a leading cause of pregnancy-related death during the first trimester. Fortunately, the rate of death from ectopic pregnancy has been declining markedly. The decrease is primarily the result of earlier diagnosis before tubal rupture, which is made possible by the availability of sensitive and specific radioimmunoassays for β-human chorionic gonadotropin (HCG), high-resolution ultrasonography, and laparoscopy. Early diagnosis of unruptured ectopic pregnancy allows the use of more conservative treatment options.

The purpose of this chapter is to present an updated review of the practical management of ectopic pregnancy.

I. DIAGNOSIS

A. Symptoms

The classic symptoms of ectopic pregnancy are abdominal pain, amenorrhea, and vaginal bleeding [1]. These symptoms may be accompanied by pregnancy discomfort such as nausea, breast tenderness, and frequent

225

urination, and in cases of tubal rupture, severe abdominal pain, light-headedness, or shock might be encountered. However, more than 50% of women are asymptomatic before tubal rupture. Ectopic pregnancy should be suspected in any women of reproductive age with these symptoms, especially those who have risk factors for an extrauterine pregnancy [1]. The risk factors are tubal pathology, previous ectopic pregnancy, previous tubal surgery, in utero diethylstilbestrol (DES) exposure, previous pelvic infection, and multiple sexual partners. Smoking, vaginal douching, infertility, pregnancy after in vitro fertilisation (IVF), and failure of tubal sterilization also increase the risk of ectopic pregnancy.

B. Physical Examination

Physical examination is often unremarkable in women with a small, unruptured ectopic pregnancy. However, vital signs may show orthostatic changes and, occasionally, fever. Other findings may include adnexal and/or abdominal tenderness, an adnexal mass, and uterine enlargement.

C. Ultrasound

Transvaginal ultrasound (TVUS) findings in conjunction with serial serum β-HCG concentrations facilitate the diagnosis of early ectopic pregnancy, permitting a more conservative treatment [2,3]. Women with risk factors for EP and those who conceived after IVF should be monitored as soon as their first missed menses. The diagnosis can then be established by laboratory and imaging studies, possibly before the occurrence of any symptoms.

Transvaginal Ultrasound

Ultrasound is most useful for identifying an intrauterine gestation. Negative ultrasound (i.e., no intrauterine or extrauterine pregnancy) does not exclude the diagnosis of EP. A heterotopic pregnancy (concomitant extrauterine and intrauterine gestation) occurs in 1 of 30,000 spontaneous conceptions; therefore the identification of an intrauterine pregnancy effectively excludes the possibility of an EP in almost all cases. However, pregnancies conceived with IVF are an exception, because the incidence of heterotopic pregnancy is as high as 1 of 100 to 1 of 3000 pregnancies [4].

The correlation between β-HCG levels and the visibility of the gestational sac is of diagnostic importance. A gestational sac may be observed by TVUS in patients with β-HCG concentration as low as 800 IU/l and is usually identified by expert ultrasonographers at concentration above 1500 IU/l [5]. The absence of an intrauterine gestational sac at β-HCG above 1500 IU/l strongly suggests an EP. Ultrasound may also demonstrate free fluid within the peritoneal cavity, suggesting an intra-abdominal bleeding. This finding strongly suggests an ectopic pregnancy when no intrauterine gestation is observed, although the blood could also be coming from a hemorrhagic cyst.

Using both TVUS and color-Doppler technology can increase the sensitivity of detecting an ectopic pregnancy. Ectopic pregnancies are characterized by the combined findings of an adnexal mass and peritrophoblastic flow on color Doppler. Blood flow in the fallopian tube containing EP is 20–45% higher than in the opposite tube [6]. However, the use of TVUS and HCG measurement is usually sufficient in establishing the diagnosis in clinical practice.

D. β-HCG

Serum β-HCG can be detected as early as 8 days after the luteinizing hormone (LH) surge, if pregnancy has occurred. The β-HCG concentration in normal intrauterine gestation rises in a curvilinear fashion until 41 days of gestation, at which time it plateaus at approximately 100,000 IU/l and the mean doubling time for the hormones is from 1.4 to 2.1 days [7,8]. As an example, studies in viable intrauterine pregnancies have demonstrated that in 85% of these gestations the β-HCG concentration rises by at least 66% every 48 days during the first 40 days of pregnancy; and in only 15% of viable pregnancies the rate of rise is less than this threshold. The rate of rise is normally slow after 40 days of pregnancy, but by this time an intrauterine pregnancy should be visible on transvaginal ultrasound examination.

The β-HCG concentration rises at much slower rate in most, but not all, ectopic and nonviable intrauterine gestations. There is a 10–15% interassay variability in these measurements, as well as variability between laboratories. Therefore, interpretation of serial β-HCG concentration is more reliable when assays are performed in the same laboratory.

E. Curettage

Trophoblastic tissue obtained by uterine curettage will distinguish between an intrauterine pregnancy and an EP. However, the use of curettage as a diagnostic tool is limited by the potential for disruption of a viable pregnancy [2]. In addition, chorionic villi are not detected by histopathology in 20% of curettage specimens from elective termination of pregnancy [9].

Some authors have recommended curettage in women with HCG concentration below the discriminatory zone and with a low doubling rate to distinguish between a nonviable intrauterine pregnancy and an EP, thus avoiding unnecessary methotrexate (MTX) administration [10]. However, it is more practical and less invasive to continue observation or administer one dose of methotrexate than to perform curettage. The side effects of one dose of methotrexate are negligible.

F. Laparoscopy

Laparoscopy is rarely required for diagnostic purposes only; transvaginal ultrasound examination and β-HCG measurements are usually sufficient for diagnosis. However, an ectopic pregnancy detected at laparoscopy should be treated immediately by surgery.

II. DIAGNOSTIC EVALUATION

Following history and physical examination, the diagnostic evaluation of a woman with suspected EP begins with determination of the β-HCG concentration and a transvaginal sonogram.

A. β-HCG Levels > 1500 IU/l

The interpretation of a β-HCG concentration at this level depends upon the findings on TVUS.

Positive Ultrasound

Presence of an intrauterine pregnancy almost always excludes the presence of an EP. Fetal cardiac activity, a gestational sac with a clear fetal pole, or yolk sac in an extrauterine location is diagnostic of an EP.

Negative Ultrasound

An EP is very likely in the absence of an intrauterine pregnancy on TVUS when serum β-HCG concentration is >1500 IU/l. However, there is no known discriminatory level for twin gestations and there is variability in the level of expertise among ultrasonographers. For these reasons, the next step is to confirm the diagnostic impression by repeating the TVUS examination and β-HCG measurements 2–3 days later. The diagnosis of EP is certain at this time if an intrauterine pregnancy is not observed on TVUS and the serum β-HCG concentration is not increasing or plateaued.

A falling β-HCG concentration is most consistent with a failed pregnancy (e.g., arrested pregnancy, blighted ovum, tubal abortion, and spontaneously resolving EP). The rate of fall is slower with an EP than with a complete abortion. Weekly β-HCG concentrations should be monitored until the result is negative for pregnancy.

B.   β-HCG levels >1500 IU/l and an Adnexal Mass

An extrauterine pregnancy is almost certain when the serum β-HCG concentration is >1500 IU/l, a nonspecific adnexal mass (i.e., without evidence of an embryo or yolk sac) is present, and no intrauterine pregnancy is observed on TVUS.

C.   β-HCG <1500 IU/l

A serum β-HCG of <1500 IU/l with a TVUS examination that is negative should be followed by repetition of both of these tests in 3 days to follow the rate of rise of the HCG. Serum β-HCG concentrations usually double every 1.5–2 days until 6–7 weeks of gestation in viable intrauterine pregnancies (and in some ectopic gestations). A β-HCG concentration that does not double over 72 hours, associated with a TVUS examination that does not show an intrauterine gestation, means that the pregnancy is nonviable, such as an ectopic gestation or intrauterine pregnancy that is destined to abort. The clinician can be certain that a normal intrauterine pregnancy is not present and can administer medical treatment.

A normally rising β-HCG concentration should be evaluated with TVUS until an intrauterine pregnancy or an ectopic pregnancy can be demonstrated. A falling β-HCG concentration is most consistent with a failed pregnancy: either an EP or an arrested pregnancy.

III. MEDICAL MANAGEMENT WITH METHOTREXATE

Medical treatment of EP with MTX is one of the most important developments in the management of this disorder. This conservative approach has supplanted surgical therapy in most cases [2,3,10–13]. The success rate in properly selected women is 86–94% [3].

A. Indications for MTX

The most successful candidates for MTX treatment are women who have

An asymptomatic ectopic pregnancy;
Ability and willingness to comply with post-treatment monitoring;
Serum β-HCG concentration of <5000 IU/l before treatment; and
Tubal size of <3 cm and no fetal cardiac activity on ultrasonographic examination.

A high serum β-HCG concentration is the most important factor associated with treatment failure [10,11]. In a series of 350 women treated with a single dose of MTX, the mean HCG concentration was significantly lower in women with successful treatment compared to those in whom the therapy failed (4019 IU/l versus 13,420 IU/l, respectively) [3]. In another smaller study, the failure rates when the initial serum β-HCG level was greater than or less than 4000 IU/l were 65 and 7.5%, respectively [12].

B. Contraindications to MTX

Some women are not appropriate candidates for medical therapy and should be managed surgically [2]. Those who are hemodynamically unstable, not likely to be compliant with post-therapeutic monitoring, and who do not have timely access to medical institution should be treated surgically. The presence of fetal cardiac activity is a relative contraindication to medical treatment. In addition, women with a high baseline HCG concentration (>5000 IU/l) are more likely to require multiple courses of medical therapy or experience treatment failure; they may be better served by conservative laparoscopic surgery [13].

C. Pretreatment Evaluation

All patients should have a complete history and physical examination prior to initiation of treatment, and pretreatment testing should include baseline β-HCG, complete blood count, blood group determination, liver and renal function tests, and transvaginal ultrasound.

D. Single-Dose MTX

The most practical approach to therapy is administration of a single intramuscular dose of MTX (50 mg/m^2 of body surface area [BSA]) [14]. A body surface area calculator may be used to determine the BSA; alternatively, BSA can be calculated based upon height and weight on the day of treatment.

Rhogam should be administrated if the woman is Rh (D)-negative and the blood group of her male partner is Rh (D)-positive or unknown.

E. Side Effects

Adverse reactions to MTX are usually mild and self-limiting. The most common are stomatitis and conjunctivitis. Rare side effects include gastritis, enteritis, dermatitis, pleuritis, alopecia, elevated liver enzymes, and bone marrow suppression.

F. Monitoring and Evaluation

Measurement of serum β-HCG concentration and ultrasound examination should be performed weekly. An increase in β-HCG levels in the 3 days following therapy (i.e., up to day 4) and mild abdominal pain of short duration (1–2 days) are common. The pain may be due to tubal abortion or tubal distention from hematoma formation and usually can be controlled with nonsteroidal anti-inflammatory drugs. The EP is often observed to increase in size and may persist for weeks on serial ultrasound examination [15]. This probably represents hematoma, rather than persistent trophoblastic tissue.

Occasionally, pain may be severe, but most women with severe pain do not need surgical intervention. For example, a review of 56 women with abdominal pain severe enough to be evaluated in the clinic or emergency room or requiring hospitalization found that only eight patients subsequently required surgery [16]. Hemodynamically stable women should be observed closely, however, because severe pain is one sign of tubal rupture necessitating surgery.

A second dose of MTX should be administrated if the serum β-HCG concentration on day 7 has not declined by at least 25% from the day 0 level. Approximately 20% of women will require a second dose of MTX [17]. The β-HCG concentration usually declines to less than 15 IU/l by 35 days post-injection, but may take as long as 109 days [17]. Weekly assays should be obtained until this level is reached. The protocol for methotrexate treatment is depicted in Table 1 [2].

G. Multidose MTX

Multiple-dose MTX regimens with folinic acid rescue were initially administered for treatment of interstitial ectopic pregnancy [18]. Single-dose MTX therapy is less expensive, has fewer side effects, requires less intensive monitoring, and does not require folinic acid. The overall rate of resolution of EP reported in the literature is greater than 90% for both single-dose and multiple-doses protocols [17].

Table 1 Protocol of Methotrexate Treatment for Ectopic Pregnancy

Pretreatment tests	Complete blood count
	Blood group and titer
	Liver and renal function tests
	Serum β-HCG
	Transvaginal ultrasound
Treatment day (day 0)	Methotrexate injection intramuscularly (i.m.)
	Rhogam 300 μg i.m. if needed
	Discontinue folinic acid supplements
	Advise the patient to refrain from strenuous exercise and sexual intercourse
Day 4	Serum β-HCG
Day 7	Serum β-HCG
	Transvaginal ultrasound
	Second dose of methotrexate if the decline in serum β-HCG is <25% than day 0 level
Weekly	Serum β-HCG until the level is <10 mIU/ml
	Transvaginal ultrasound
Any time	Laparoscopy if ultrasound reveals hemoperitoneum of >100 ml, severe abdominal pain, or acute abdomen

H. Local MTX

MTX, hyperosmolar glucose, potassium chloride, and prostaglandin F2-alpha are agents that can be locally injected into the ectopic gestational sac under ultrasound guidance. In one study, the immediate outcome of local MTX administration in selected cases appeared similar to that with laparoscopic salpingostomy [19]. However, the long-term outcome was better with local MTX treatment: higher subsequent pregnancy rates and lower recurrent EP rates were achieved than with surgical therapy. It is not known whether these benefits were treatment-dependent or related to baseline tubal status.

Local treatment, however, is highly operator dependent ultrasonographically and not practical when performed laparoscopically. Women bearing the costs and risks of laparoscopic surgery should have definitive treatment (i.e., removal of the ectopic gestation) at the time of the procedure.

IV. MEDICAL VERSUS SURGICAL TREATMENT

Several randomized studies have shown that medical treatment of selected cases of EP is as effective as laparoscopic treatment [20–22]. As an example, a meta-analysis reported mean success rates for MTX and laparoscopic therapy of 87 and 91%, respectively [23]. Complication rates for medical therapy averaged 10% for minor complications (e.g., tubal rupture during follow-up), whereas complication rates for laparoscopy were 2% for intraoperative complications and 9% for postoperative complications. Both treatments appear to be equally effective for preserving tubal patency [21]. However, the time required for β-HCG concentrations to reach undetectable levels is faster after laparoscopic surgery, thus reducing the period of post-treatment monitoring.

Medical treatment may have a negative impact on the woman's quality of life [24]. For example, some women experience anxiety and emotional distress related to the initial rise in serum β-HCG concentration, abdominal pain occurring after medical treatment, prolonged vaginal bleeding, the risk of tubal rupture present during therapy, the lengthy period of post-treatment monitoring, and the possible need for a second course of MTX. A detailed informed consent reviewing the procedure, monitoring, outcome, risks, and benefits of both medical and surgical therapy should be fully discussed with the patient before administration of MTX.

V. SURGICAL TREATMENT

Management of EP has dramatically changed from a primarily surgical approach to the medical therapies, which currently predominate [2,3]. However, some women are not good candidates for medical therapy and undergo surgical therapy by choice or necessity.

A. Indications for Surgery

Surgery should only be performed if a TVUS shows a tubal ectopic pregnancy or an adnexal mass suggestive of ectopic pregnancy. If an abnormality is not imaged ultrasonographically, there is a high probability that an EP will not be visualized at surgery. Therefore, these women should be managed conservatively with either medical therapy or expectant management. Repeating the ultrasound examination after a few days may localize an abnormality, thus enabling a surgical procedure if this option is desired.

Specific indications for surgical therapy include:

Ruptured ectopic pregnancy, especially in a hemodynamically unstable woman.

Inability or unwillingness to comply with post-treatment monitoring after medical therapy.

Lack of timely access to a medical institution for management of tubal rupture, which can occur during conservative therapy.

Women with a serum β-HCG concentration >5000 mIU/ml before treatment, tubal size >3 cm, or fetal cardiac activity on ultrasonographic examination are more likely to experience treatment failure with MTX.

B. Type of Surgical Procedures

Laparotomy vs. Laparoscopy

Three prospective, randomized trials including a total of 231 women compared laparotomy to laparoscopy and found that laparoscopic conservative surgery was superior to laparotomy [25–27]. The overall findings from these studies were

The laparoscopic approach resulted in less blood loss, lower analgesic requirements, and shorter duration of hospital stay.

Laparoscopy yielded significant cost savings per patient.

The reproductive outcome after salpingostomy by either approach was similar. Sixty-nine women in the laparoscopy group and 76 in the laparotomy group desired future pregnancy; the rate of subsequent intrauterine pregnancy for each group was 61 and 53%, respectively. The rates of repeat ectopic pregnancy following salpingostomy by laparoscopy or laparotomy were 7 and 14%, respectively.

Most ectopic pregnancies, even in the presence of hemoperitoneum, heterotopic pregnancy, and interstitial pregnancy, can be treated by a laparoscopic procedure. The surgical approach depends upon the experience and judgment of the surgeon.

Salpingostomy vs. Salpingectomy

The intrauterine pregnancy and recurrent EP rates reported after salpingostomy are 61 and 15%, respectively [3]. By comparison, the intrauterine pregnancy rate after salpingectomy is only 38%. These differences likely reflect tubal status at surgery, rather than the choice of surgical procedure. However, in the absence of a randomized study, salpingostomy is the preferred treatment of EP in women who are hemodynamically stable and wish to preserve their fertility [2,3].

Indications for Salpingectomy

Some ectopic pregnancies are best treated by salpingectomy, instead of salpingostomy. These conditions include: uncontrolled bleeding from the implantation side; recurrent ectopic pregnancy in the same tube; severely damaged tube; large tubal pregnancy (i.e., greater than 5 cm); and women who have completed childbearing. In these situations, there is a low probability of future normal tubal function and the risk of persistent or recurrent tubal problems is high.

C. Surgical Technique

Laparoscopic Salpingostomy

Linear salpingostomy is considered the gold standard for management of EP in women who wish to preserve their fertility.

The EP is identified and the tube is immobilized with laparoscopic forceps [28]. A 22-gauge needle is inserted through a 5-mm portal and used to inject a solution of vasopressin (0.2 IU/ml of physiologic saline) into the wall of the tube at the area of maximal distention; this helps to minimize bleeding at the salpingostomy site. Using laser, unipolar needle electrocautery, or scissors, the surgeon makes a 10- to 15-mm longitudinal incision along the antimesenteric border overlying the

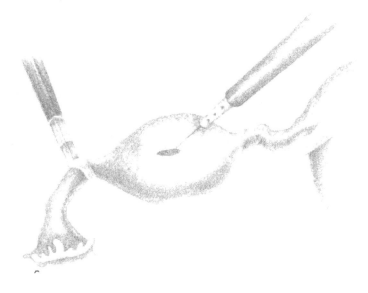

Figure 1   Linear salpingostomy: injection of vasopressin into the wall of the tube. (Courtesy of Tulandi's Atlas of Laparoscopic and Hysteroscopic Techniques for Gynecologists, 2nd ed. London: WB Saunders, 1999.)

ectopic (Figs. 1–3). The products of conception are flushed out of the tube using a combination of hydrodissection with irrigating solution under high pressure and gentle blunt dissection with a suction irrigator. The specimen can then be grasped with a 10-mm claw forceps to remove it from the abdominal cavity or grasped with a laparoscopic pouch.

The tube is carefully irrigated and inspected under water for hemostasis. Bleeding points can be controlled by pressure or coagulated with light application of bipolar coagulation. If bleeding persists, vessels in the mesosalpinx can be ligated with a 6-0 polyglactin suture.

The placental bed inside the tube should not be coagulated because this will seriously damage the tube. The incision is left open to heal by secondary intention; the subsequent rates of fertility and adhesion formation are similar after primary closure or secondary intention [29].

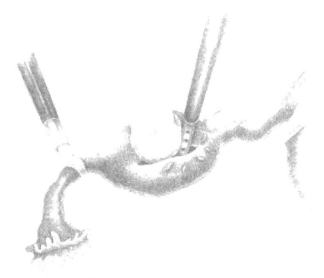

Figure 2   A longitudinal incision is made on the antemesosalpinx of the tube. (Courtesy of Tulandi's Atlas of Laparoscopic and Hysteroscopic Techniques for Gynecologists, 2nd ed. London: WB Saunders, 1999.)

Laparoscopic Salpingectomy

There are several methods for total laparoscopic salpingectomy. One approach is to bring the fallopian tube through a pretied surgical loop using a grasping forceps. The knot is tightened and the tube is resected and removed. Another approach is by coagulating the tube proximal and distal to the ectopic gestation.

VI.   EXPECTANT MANAGEMENT

Expectant management of ectopic pregnancy is not a new concept. In one older series of 114 hospitalized patients with a typical ectopic pregnancy, 57 were safely managed expectantly, without surgical or medical intervention (except narcotics) [30]. A review of 10 studies that prospectively examined the efficacy of expectant management found an overall efficacy of approximately 70% [3]. This approach appears

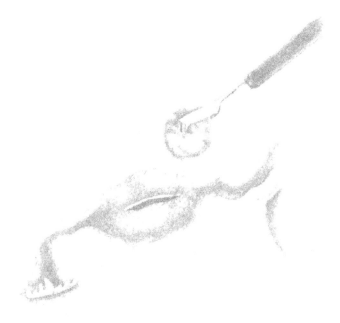

Figure 3 By using a suction irrigator, the products of conception are flushed out of the tube. (Courtesy of Tulandi's Atlas of Laparoscopic and Hysteroscopic Techniques for Gynecologists, 2nd ed. London: WB Saunders, 1999.)

reasonable based upon data from one series that followed 135 women with unknown location of their pregnancy [31].

The role of expectant management in women with known EP is limited due to an unacceptable risk of rupture when compared to the high efficacy, safety, and accessibility of medical or surgical treatment. Medical treatment, primarily with MTX, is the preferred alternative to surgical therapy of EP. Expectant management is a less desirable option.

VII. PERSISTENT ECTOPIC PREGNANCY

Persistent ectopic pregnancy occurs more often after laparoscopy than laparotomy, 8 vs. 4%, respectively [2]. However, this could be a reflection of the surgeon's expertise and experience.

A.   Prevention of Persistent Ectopic Pregnancy

Persistent trophoblast is typically found proximal to the tubal gestation; therefore, attention should be directed to this area. Removing the products of conception piecemeal with forceps may lead to retained trophoblastic tissue. Flushing the gestational products out of the tube using suction irrigation under pressure might be helpful.

B.   Diagnosis and Treatment of Persistent Ectopic Pregnancy

The clearance rate of serum β-HCG following salpingostomy is similar to that after salpingectomy: the postoperative day 1 serum β-HCG generally declines by more than 50% of the preoperative value [32]. Many authors recommend weekly serum β-HCG measurements after laparoscopic salpingostomy. The incidence of persistent EP in our hands is extremely low; therefore we perform a single β-HCG measurement 1 week after surgery. A level less than 5% of the preoperative value is consistent with complete resolution of the EP; a higher value calls for repeat measurement 1 week later. Treatment is administered if the level does not decline.

A single dose of MTX (50 mg/m^2 intramuscularly) is administered to women with persistent EP. Transvaginal ultrasound examination and measurement of serum β-HCG concentration are performed weekly until the level is less than 10 mIU/ml.

VIII.   REPRODUCTIVE PERFORMANCE AFTER AN ECTOPIC PREGNANCY

Many factors in addition to the type of surgical procedure influence a woman's fertility rate after a tubal pregnancy [33–38].

A history of prior infertility is the most important factor for subsequent fertility [34]. For example, the pregnancy rate following ectopic pregnancy in women with a history of infertility is one-fourth that of normal women [34].

Prior tubal damage is associated with a decreased pregnancy rate

compared to controls with normal-appearing tubes, 42 and 79%, respectively [35].
Ipsilateral periadnexal adhesions reflect poor condition of the tube [36].

IX. CONCLUSIONS

Early diagnosis has allowed conservative surgical and medical management of ectopic pregnancy. The clinical presentation, serum β-HCG concentrations and transvaginal ultrasound findings dictate the management of this condition. Medical treatment with methotrexate can be given to women with asymptomatic ectopic pregnancy, have high compliance, serum β-HCG <5000 mIU/ml, tubal size <3 cm, and no fetal cardiac activity on ultrasound. The most practical and efficient method is a single intramuscular injection of methotrexate. Those who do not meet the criteria for MTX treatment should be treated surgically, and the best alternative for women who wish to preserve their fertility is laparoscopic salpingostomy. Persistent ectopic pregnancy is found in about 5% of cases after surgery, and this can be treated with methotrexate.

REFERENCES

1. Ankum WM, Mol BWJ, Van Der Veen F, Bossuyt PMM. Risk factors for ectopic pregnancy: a meta-analysis. Fertil Steril 1996; 65:1093–1099.
2. Tulandi T. Current protocol for ectopic pregnancy. Contemp Obstet Gynecol 1999; 44:42–55.
3. Yao M, Tulandi T. Current status of surgical and non-surgical management of ectopic pregnancy. Fertil Steril 1997; 67:421–433.
4. Molloy D, Deambrosis W, Keeping D, Hynes J, Harrison K, Hennessey J. Multiple-sited (heterotopic) pregnancy after in vitro fertilization and gamete intrafallopian transfer. Fertil Steril 1990; 53:1068–1071.
5. Paul M, Schaff E, Nichols M. The roles of clinical assessment, human chorionic gonadotropin assays, and ultrasonography in medical abortion practice. Am J Obstet Gynecol 2000; 183:S34–S43.

6. Kirchler HC, Seebacher S, Alge AA, Muller-Holzner E, Fessler S, Kolle D. Early diagnostis of tubal pregnancy: changes in tubal blood flow evaluated by endovaginal color Doppler sonography. Obstet Gynecol 1993; 82:561–565.

7. Daya S. Human chorionic gonadotrophin increases in normal early pregnancy. Am J Obstet Gynecol 1987; 156:286–290.

8. Kadar N, DeCherney AH, Romero R. Receiver operating characteristic (ROC) curve analysis of the relative efficacy of single and serial chorionic gonadotrophin determinations in the early diagnosis of ectopic pregnancy. Fertil Steril 1982; 37:542–547.

9. Lindahl B, Ahlgren M. Identification of chorion villi in abortion specimens. Obstet Gynecol 1986; 67:79–81.

10. Lipscomb GH, McCord ML, Stovall TG, Huff G, Portera SG, Ling FW. Predictors of success of methotrexate treatment in women with tubal ectopic pregnancies. N Engl J Med 1999; 341:1974–1978.

11. Lipscomb GH, Stovall TG, Ling FW. Nonsurgical treatment of ectopic pregnancy. N Engl J Med 2000: 343:1325–1329.

12. Tawfiq A, Agameya A, Claman P. Predictors of treatment failure for ectopic pregnancy treated with single-dose methotrexate. Fertil Steril 2000; 74:877–880.

13. Hajenius PJ, Mol BWJ, Bossuyt PMM, et al. Interventions for tubal ectopic pregnancy. Cochrane Database Syst Rev 2000; CD000324.

14. Stovall TG, Ling FW. Single-dose methotrexate: an expanded clinical trial. Am J Obstet Gynecol 1993; 168:1759–1762.

15. Brown DL, Felker RE, Stovall TG, Emerson DS, Ling FW. Serial endovaginal sonography of ectopic pregnancies treated with methotrexate. Obstet Gynecol 1991; 77:406–409.

16. Lipscomb GH, Puckett KJ, Bran D, Ling FW. Management of separation pain after single-dose methotrexate therapy for ectopic pregnancy. Obstet Gynecol 1999; 93:590–593.

17. Lipscomb GH, Bran D, McCord ML, Portera JC, Ling FW. Analysis of three hundred fifteen ectopic pregnancies treated with single-dose methotrexate. Am J Obstet Gynecol 1998; 178:1354–1358.

18. Tanaka T, Hayashi H, Kutsuzawa T, Fujimoro S, Ichinoe K. Treatment of interstitial ectopic pregnancy with methotrexate: report of a successful case. Fertil Steril 1982; 37:851–852.

19. Fernandez H, Yves Vincent SC, Pauthier S, Audibert F, Frydman R. Randomized trial of conservative laparoscopic treatment and methotrexate administration in ectopic pregnancy and subsequent fertility. Hum Reprod 1998; 13:3239–3243.

20. Saraj AJ, Wilcox JG, Najmabadi S, Stein SM, Johnson MB, Paulson RJ. Resolution of hormional markers of ectopic gestation: a randomized trial comparing single-dose intramuscular methotrexate with salpingostomy. Obstet Gynecol 1998; 92:989–994.

21. Hajenius PJ, Engelsbel S, Mol BW, van der Veen F, Ankum WM, Bossuyt PM, Hemrika DJ, Lammes FB. Randomized trial of systemic methotrexate versus laparoscopic salpingostomy in tubal pregnancy. Lancet 1997; 350:774–779.

22. Sowter MC, Farquhar CM, Petrie KJ, Gudex G. A randomized trial comparing single-dose systemic methotrexate and laparoscopic surgery for the treatment of unruptured tubal pregnancy. Fertil Steril 2001; 108: 192–203.

23. Morlock RJ, Lafata JE, Eisenstein D. Cost-effectiveness of single-dose methotrexate compared with laparoscopic treatment of ectopic pregnancy. Obstet Gynecol 2000; 95:407–412.

24. Nieuwerk PT, Hajenius PJ, Ankum WM, van der Veen F, Wijker W, Bossuyt PM. Systemic methotrexate therapy versus laparoscopic salpingostomy in patients with tubal pregnancy. Part I. Impact on patient's health-related quality of life. Fertil Steril 1998; 70:511–517.

25. Murphy AA, Kettel LM, Nager CW, Wujek JJ, Torp VA, Chin HG. Operative laparoscopy versus laparotomy for the management of ectopic pregnancy: a prospective trial. Fertil Steril 1992; 57:1180–1185.

26. Vermesh M, Silva PD, Rosen GF, Stein AL, Fossum GT, Souer MV. Management of unruptured ectopic gestation by linear salpingostomy: a prospective, randomized clinical trial of laparoscopy versus laparotomy. Obstet Gynecol 1989; 73:400–404.

27. Lundorff P, Thorburn J, Hahlin M, Kalfelt B, Lindblom B. Laparoscopic surgery in ectopic pregnancy: a randomized trial versus laparotomy. Acta Obstet Gynecol Scand 1991; 70:343–348.

28. Tulandi T. Tubal ectopic pregnancy: salpingostomy and salpingectomy. In: Tulandi T, ed. Atlas of Laparoscopy and Hysteroscopy Techniques. London: W. B. Saunders, 1999: 49–57.

29. Tulandi T, Guralnick M. Treatment of tubal ectopic pregnancy by salpingotomy with or without tubal suturing and salpingectomy. Fertil Steril 1991; 55:53–55.

30. Lund J. Early ectopic pregnancy. J Obstet Gynecol Br Emp 1955; 62: 70.

31. Banerjee S, Aslam N, Zosmer N, Woelfer B, Jurkovic D. The expectant management of women with early pregnancy of unknown location. Ultrasound Obstet Gynecol 1999; 14:231–236.

32. Spandorfer SD, Sawin SW, Benjamin I, Barnhart KT. Postoperative day 1 serum human chorionic gonadotropin level as predictor of persistent ectopic pregnancy after conservative surgical management. Fertil Steril 1997; 68:430-434.

33. Ory SJ, Nnadi E, Herrmann R, O'Brien PS, Melron LJ III. Fertility after ectopic pregnancy. Fertil Steril 1993; 60:231–235.

34. Sultana CJ, Easley K, Collins RL. Outcome of laparoscopic versus traditional surgery for ectopic pregnancies. Fertil Steril 1992; 57:285–289.

35. Silva PD, Schaper AM, Rooney B. Reproductive outcome after 143 laparoscopic procedures foe ectopic pregnancy. Obstet Gynecol 1993; 81:710–715.

36. Pouly JL, Chapron C, Manhes H, Canis M, Wattiez A, Bruhar MA. Multifactoral analysis of fertility after conservative laparoscopic treatment of ectopic pregnancy in a series of 223 patients. Fertil Steril 1991; 56:453–460.

37. Ego A, Subtil D, Cosson M, Legoueff F, Houfflin-Debarge V, Querdeu D. Survival analysis of fertility after ectopic pregnancy. Fertil Steril 2001; 75:560–566.

38. Dubuisson JB, Aubriot FX, Foulot H, Bruel D, Bouquet de Joliniere J, Mandelbrot L. Reproductive outcome after laparoscopic salpingectomy for tubal pregnancy. Fertil Steril 1990; 53:1004–1007.

11

Laparoscopic Surgery for Pelvic Pain

Christopher Sutton
Royal Surrey County Hospital and University of Surrey, Guildford, Surrey, England

The introduction of laparoscopy heralded a new era in gynecological practice, replacing art with science and taking the guesswork out of the diagnosis of many pelvic and abdominal ailments. Laparoscopy is not only important in making a diagnosis but is increasingly employed in the surgical treatment of women who present with pelvic pain.

I. PELVIC PAIN IN WOMEN OF REPRODUCTIVE AGE

The only community-based study on the frequency of this complaint comes from the United States, where Mathias et al. [1] quoted a prevalence rate of 15%, and in addition to the medical costs associated with hospital attendances and treatment, the economic assessment of the problem showed that 15% of the employed women reported time lost from work and 45% reported reduced productivity.

Because the diagnosis of a condition such as endometriosis carries significant health implications for any woman, it is important that the diagnostic laparoscopy is performed by an experienced gynecologist. It is also important that laparoscopy is only performed after a thorough multidisciplinary diagnostic evaluation has been carried out. Certain conditions, such as adenomyosis, cannot reliably be diagnosed at laparoscopy and require more expensive investigations, such as magnetic resonance imaging (MRI) and directed myometrial biopsies and, even then, the diagnosis is often made retrospectively after the uterus has been removed at hysterectomy.

In an excellent review of the published literature, Porpora and Gomel [2] showed that a disease entity is encountered at laparoscopy in more than 60% of patients with chronic pelvic pain, but in only 28% of those without chronic pelvic pain. It would appear that laparoscopy is the gold standard in the diagnosis of a cause for pelvic pain compared with physical examination. Vercellini et al. [3] found abnormalities at laparoscopy in 79 of the 126 patients studied, who had a completely normal physical examination. The incidence of the pathology detected when laparoscopy is performed for the diagnosis of pelvic pain varies widely between 16 and 33% for endometriosis and from 23 to 40% for adhesions, and negative findings can be encountered in between 15 and 30% of diagnostic procedures [4–7]. Much of this discrepancy can be explained by different types of referral practice and the increased sophistication in recognizing the more subtle or atypical forms of endometriosis. New developments in conscious pelvic pain mapping have shown that the relationship between pelvic pain and the laparoscopic findings are not always clear, and it does not necessarily follow that the discovery of a lesion is the cause of the presenting pain. Nevertheless, some of the principle diagnostic conditions discovered can be treated by laparoscopic surgery at the same time as the diagnosis is made; these conditions will be discussed in the order of their prevalence.

II. ENDOMETRIOSIS

Endometriosis is a strange and increasingly common condition and the precise pathogenesis of the disease is still unclear. Although most patients present with severe dysmenorrhea, deep dyspareunia, infertility, and pelvic pain (unrelated to the menstrual cycle), it is surprising that in O'Connor's classic monologue, reporting his lifetime experience with the disease, he found 22% of patients diagnosed at laparoscopy were completely asymptomatic [8]. The severity of the pain and other symptoms has no relation to the stage of the disease [9] on the revised American Fertility Society (AFS) scale. Pain can be caused by the production of certain prostaglandins, particularly prostaglandin F [10], and even small lesions are capable of producing this pain-mediating hormone in large amounts, which accounts for the finding that patients with mild or minimal disease can often have more pain that those with extensive disease, which is often found incidentally at laparotomy for a pelvic mass in an otherwise asymptomatic patient. There is, however, a positive correlation between severe pelvic pain and deep infiltrating endometriosis [11]. This is particularly the case when the disease involves the rectovaginal septum or the uterosacral ligaments, where pain is induced by infiltration, expansion (fibromuscular hyperplasia), and tissue damage among the nerve fibers of the Lee-Frankenhäuser plexus [12]. It is important to realize, however, that the appearances of this deep infiltration can often only be recognized by the experienced and discerning eye of a specialist in the treatment of endometriosis, and others, sadly, would pronounce this a normal pelvis (Fig. 1) because most of the abnormal infiltrating tissue can be palpated deep in the posterior or lateral fornix rather than be seen.

Some authorities [13] regard peritoneal implants, ovarian endometriomas, and deep infiltrating disease as three completely separate conditions, the latter being a manifestation of adenomyosis externa [14]. They will therefore be considered separately in the following sections.

III. LAPAROSCOPIC SURGERY

Laparoscopic surgery was deservedly hailed as a revolution of surgical practice, but it is a shame that the early enthusiasts, myself included, concentrated on the immediate advantages to the patient in terms of short hospital stay and lowered morbidity, and only presented their results in terms of retrospective studies. Because the evolution of these techniques largely occurred in non-university hospitals, it is not surprising that academic colleagues in the teaching hospitals regarded pain improvement statistics following laparoscopic ablation of peritoneal endometriosis with grave suspicion and demanded solid evidence in the form of a prospective, randomized, controlled trial. Although many

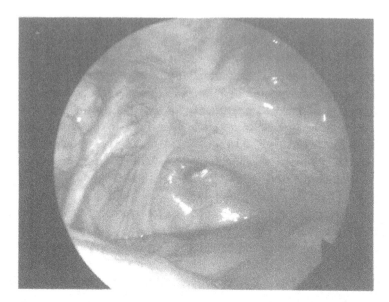

Figure 1 Extensive scarring of the right uterosacral ligament and infiltration laterally toward the left ureter. The central dimple in the posterior cul-de-sac indicates retraction from a nodule in the rectovaginal septum, which can be felt by deep palpation, both vaginally and rectally, rather than seen.

centers have attempted prospective cohort studies there is only one trial in the current literature that is not only randomized and prospective, but compares laser treatment against expectant (sham) management alone, and has the added advantage of being double blind. Because the relief of pain is prone to subjective bias and operator enthusiasm, the study remains unique and will be described in detail.

IV. EVIDENCE-BASED MEDICINE—THE GUILDFORD LASER LAPAROSCOPY TRIAL (GRADE A EVIDENCE)

The aim of this study was to assess the efficacy of laser laparoscopy by the established scientific method of a prospective, randomized, double-blind, controlled trial, comparing the results of those women with minimal to moderate endometriosis (AFS stages I to III) [15] who were treated by the laser ablation of peritoneal deposits and those in the sham arm who had diagnostic laparoscopy alone.

This study was approved by the Hospital Ethics Committee, but they reasonably felt that it was unethical to withhold treatment from patients in severe pain due to stage IV disease, particularly because our previous experience had shown 80% pain relief in this group, most of whom had failed to respond to medical therapy [16].

The study population was recruited from women seen in the gyne-cological outpatient clinic with pain suggestive of endometriosis who had been advised to undergo a diagnostic laparoscopy. To be included in the study, women were between 18 and 45 years of age, were neither pregnant nor lactating, and had not received any treatment (medical or surgical) for endometriosis in the previous 6 months. The study was explained in detail and informed consent was obtained. Before the lap-aroscopy, the patients were asked to record the intensity of their pain on a 10-cm linear analogue scale marked from 0 to 10; 0 representing no pain at all and 10 representing the worst pain they had experienced in their life [17].

Between March 1990 and February 1993, 74 women were re-cruited and at the time of laparoscopy treatment was allocated randomly (computer generated randomisation sequence) to laser treatment or ex-pectant management. The laser treatment included vaporisation of all visible endometriotic implants, adhesiolysis and uterine nerve transec-tion using a triple puncture technique. The patients in the sham arm had exactly the same incisions (three) but merely had a diagnostic lap-aroscopy, although during this it was necessary to remove the serosan-guinous fluid from the Pouch of Douglas in order to perform a thorough inspection of the entire pelvic peritoneum. Patients were not informed which treatment group they had been allocated to and were followed up at 3 months and 6 months after surgery by an independent observer (research nurse), who also was unaware of the treatment that had been carried out. She had no access to the hospital notes or operation details and therefore the study was genuinely double-blind.

A. Results of the Study

Of 74 women who entered the trial, 63 (32 laser, 31 expectant) com-pleted the study to the 6-month follow-up visit. The 11 patients who

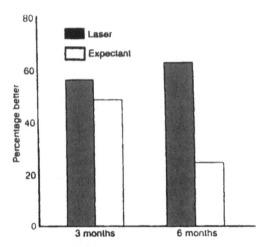

Figure 2   Proportion of patients with pain symptom alleviation at all stages.
(From Ref. 42.)

were excluded had either become pregnant or been put on the oral contraceptive by their family doctor, although both the patients and the
doctors were requested not to do this during the course of the study.
Three were lost to follow-up, all having moved overseas with no for-
warding address.

The results are shown in Figures 2 and 3 and it can clearly be
seen that at 3 months postoperation there was very little difference

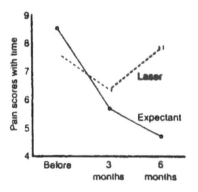

Figure 3   Median visual analogue pain scores (with time). (From Ref. 42.)

between the two groups, but at 6 months the difference reached statistical significance: 62.5% of the patients who had the laser treatment were better and only 22.6% of the patients who had no treatment said they were better. The results were worst for stage I disease and this is probably because some of the minimal changes seen in mild endometriosis could possibly be due to inflammatory changes, Walthard cell rests, or other nonspecific changes in the appearance of the peritoneum. Unfortunately, the disease could not be confirmed by biopsy because that would have acted as a cytoreductive procedure and could not truly be called expectant management. If the stage I patients were excluded, then 73.7% of patients achieved pain relief, which is very similar to the figure obtained in our retrospective study [18].

B.   Placebo Effect

There are several interesting features of this study that merit discussion. We were surprised that the results at 3 months were very similar for the laser group (56%) compared with the expectant group (48%). There was no significant difference between these two figures and we were surprised to find that almost half of the patients with no treatment claimed that they were better. This placebo effect has been noticed in another Italian study [19] where dysmenorrhea was reported to have improved in up to 30% of patients in the placebo arm comparing expectant management with gonadotropin-releasing hormone (GnRH) analogues. They found that this improvement did not last longer than 3 months, and that was exactly the same as our finding. The visual analogue scale clearly shows that at 6 months the women in the expectant arm had returned to the original score, whereas the laser-treated group had continued to improve. This has also demonstrated that it can take at least 3 months for the benefit of laparoscopic laser surgery to be noticed, so we now advise patients of this and only see them for follow-up at 6 months—seeing them before this will not give a realistic assessment of the treatment.

C.   Natural History of the Disease

Another benefit of this study was to allow us to examine the natural history of endometriosis because it is widely assumed that it is a progressive disease. We had the opportunity to look at a group of patients who had not received any treatment but had an established diagnosis, and to report the findings of the second-look laparoscopy and compare the changes in their symptoms [20]. At second-look laparoscopy, 10 cases (42%) had no change in the AFS score; 7 cases (29%) had an increased score, with 3 patients moving to a higher stage; but we were surprised to find that one-third of the patients (7 cases) had a reduced AFS score, with 3 patients moving to a lower stage. These patients had improved or resolved symptoms, whereas in the others the symptomatology was the same or had become more severe while they were waiting for laparoscopic laser surgery. This study enabled us to show that the disease does progress in the majority of patients, but in up to one-third it can regress and in a few of them it disappeared altogether. This finding has also been confirmed in studies on higher primates with experimentally induced endometriosis [21].

D. Long-Term Follow-Up of the Trial Patients

We recently had an opportunity to conduct a long-term follow-up on this cohort of patients by telephone interview with a mean time since the operation of 88.6 months (range 77–104 months) [22]. Of the 32 patients who had had a laser laparoscopy, we were able to contact 22 (68.8%). We had to remove four from the study (12.5%) because they had been taking the oral contraceptive pill which diminishes the symptoms of endometriosis, and six (18.8%) were lost to follow-up (Fig. 4a). Nevertheless, we found that 60% of the patients had continued to have satisfactory symptom relief, one was menopausal, and four needed mild analgesia only. Three of the patients had repeat laser laparoscopy for new disease in different sites, five were leading pain-free lives, and three of these had had successful pregnancies. Of those that continued to have painful symptoms, six had repeated laser laparoscopy on one or more occasions, and two had required psychiatric help (Munchausen syndrome) and required strong analgesia. Notably, of the six patients who eventually had a hysterectomy and bilateral salpingo-oophorectomy, all of them had a normal pelvis macroscopically at the time of operation and no histological evidence of endometriosis was

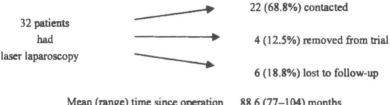

32 patients had laser laparoscopy → 22 (68.8%) contacted

→ 4 (12.5%) removed from trial

→ 6 (18.8%) lost to follow-up

Mean (range) time since operation   88.6 (77–104) months
Mean age 38.2 (33–45) years c.f.29 (18–42) years at surgery

Continued to experience   painful symptoms 9/22 (40.9%)

     6 had repeat laser laparoscopy on one or more occasions
     6 had hysterectomy (all had normal pelvis at operation)
     2 had psychiatric help and analgesia
     1 on IVF program

Satisfactory symptom relief 13/22 (59.1%) patients
     1 menopausal
     5 leading pain-free lives (3 had successful pregnancies)
     3 needed repeat laser laparoscopy for repeat disease
     4 needed mild analgesia

Figure 4   Long-term results of GLERP.

seen, apart from one very small focus of adenomyosis in one uterus (Figs. 4b and 4c).

The conclusion from this is that regardless of treatment (all of these had been taking strong medical treatment), a certain group of patients will not get better and continue to complain of pelvic pain, sadly even after a hysterectomy.

Nevertheless, laparoscopic laser surgery results in satisfactory symptom relief at 6 months and the majority of these patients continue to have symptom relief over many years. It also has the advantage that treatment can be performed at the same time as the diagnosis is made, with no extra morbidity or mortality in our experience over 18 years.

Laparoscopic laser surgery avoids the use of expensive medical treatments which often have severe and unpleasant side effects.

Although the Guildford prospective randomized controlled trial (RCT) is the only class A evidence in the Cochrane review on laparoscopic laser surgery for the treatment of pelvic pain, it has been criticized because the laser surgery not only included vaporization of the peritoneal implants and adhesiolysis where indicated, but also included laparoscopic uterine nerve ablation (LUNA) and there was justifiable concern that it may well have been the pelvic nerve ablation that had contributed to the overall good results. We have just completed a further double-blind, randomized controlled trial comparing laser ablation of peritoneal deposits plus LUNA, with laser ablation of the peritoneal deposits alone and, to our surprise, discovered that the LUNA conferred no additional benefit at all [23]. This will be further discussed at the end of the next section on pelvic denervation procedures.

V. LAPAROSCOPIC DENERVATION PROCEDURES FOR PELVIC PAIN

The perfect neuro-ablative surgical procedure for pelvic pain would interrupt all the afferent sensory nerves from all the pelvic organs and leave all other nerves unaffected. Unfortunately, this is clearly impossible because the uterus and ovaries receive their nerve supply not only through a series of anatomically distinct nervous plexuses, but also by nerves that accompany the ovarian and uterine arteries. From Figure 5, it can be seen that it would be impossible to interrupt all of these nervous pathways without damage to the vascular supply of the reproductive organs [24].

The body of the uterus appears to be innervated only by sympathetic fibers [25]. The cervix is mainly supplied by parasympathetic fibers (but also some sympathetic), which traverse the cervical division of the Lee-Frankenhäuser plexus which lies in, under, and around the attachments of the uterosacral ligament to the posterolateral aspect of the cervix [26–28]. Sympathetic fibers can also be found in this area which have reached the cervix by accompanying the uterine arteries. Excellent illustrations of Lee's original dissection showing the nerves

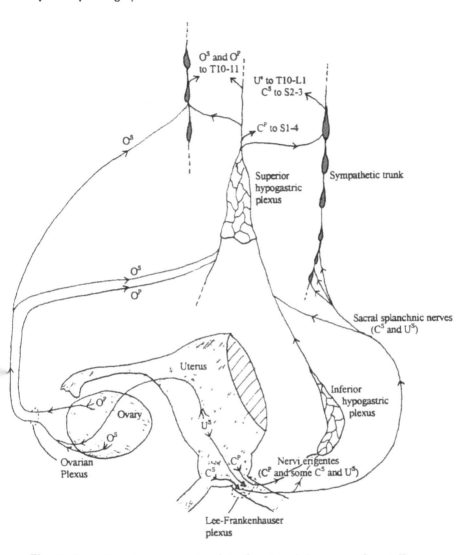

Figure 5 Afferent nerve supply of the female pelvic organs. C = Afferent nerve supply of cervix (right); O = afferent nerve supply of ovary (left); U = afferent nerve supply of uterus (right); P = parasympathetic nerve; S = sympathetic nerve.

in this plexus can be seen in the Wellcome History of Medicine Museum in London.

From the uterosacral ligaments the parasympathetic afferent fibers reach the dorsal root ganglia of the first to fourth sacral spinal nerves (S1–4) via the pelvic splanchnic nerves (nervi erigentes) and the inferior hypogastric plexus. Theoretically therefore, division of the uterosacral ligaments at the point of their attachment to the cervix should lead to interruption of most of the cervical sensory fibers and some of the corporal sensory fibers, and lead to a diminution in uterine pain at the time of menstruation. Clearly the sympathetic afferent fibers that accompany the uterine, iliac, and inferior mesenteric arteries to the sacral sympathetic trunk via the sacral splanchnic nerves will not be interrupted, and therefore complete denervation is not possible.

Surgical division of the uterosacral ligaments by LUNA or resection of the presacral nerves could be reasonably expected to diminish central pain from dysmenorrhea, but could not be expected to relieve lateral pain, especially that coming from the ovaries, because these fibers bypass the uterosacral ligament and course through the corresponding plexuses to their cells of origin in the dorsal route ganglia of the 10th and 11th thoracic spinal nerves. Indeed, some of the upper ovarian plexus afferent nerves go directly via the renal and aortic plexuses and even bypass the superior hypogastric plexus, so that even a complete presacral neurectomy would not interrupt them (Fig. 5).

A. Presacral Neurectomy

The operation of presacral neurectomy at laparotomy has been in use for at least 70 years and the first published series was in 1937 [29]. Because of the relatively high incidence of complications, this type of major abdominal surgery is rarely used currently, although, in the hands of extremely experienced and skilled laparoscopic surgeons, it can be performed laparoscopically, even on an outpatient basis. This is an extremely difficult laparoscopic procedure because the retroperitoneal space in front of the sacral promontory is extremely vascular. It is necessary to reflect the sigmoid colon laterally, aided by a left-sided tilt of the operating table, and then to coagulate all the vessels in the presacral space before dividing or excising the nerves of the superior hyper-gastric plexus. Some surgeons remove a segment of nerve to obtain histological proof of excision, whereas others merely divide the nerve (presacral neurotomy) using the potassium titanyl phosphate laser, an electrosurgical hook, or the argon beam coagulator. The nerve bundles of the superior hypogastric plexus have widely varying anatomical configurations [30] and because of the vascularity of this area bleeding, particularly from the middle sacral artery, can be extremely troublesome as also can be bleeding from the periostial blood vessels. In addition, there have been problems with certain devices, particularly the argon beam coagulator, which employs an electron channel of argon gas through which radiofrequency energy is conducted. In two operations, this energy has reflected off the surface of the periosteum and the energy has torn the common iliac vessels, resulting in catastrophic bleeding [31]. However, in skilled hands the operation can give good long-term results [32,33].

Unfortunately this procedure has a high incidence of complications, and in Chen's study, 31 of the 33 patients who underwent laparoscopic presacral neurectomy experienced constipation, which was very severe in some cases. In another study reporting presacral neurectomy at laparotomy, Candiani et al. [34] reported that 13 women had long-standing constipation, 3 had urinary urgency, and 2 had a completely painless first stage of labor. There was also one patient who required a subsequent laparotomy 48 hours postoperatively because of a presacral hematoma. Laparoscopic presacral neurectomy is regarded as an extremely advanced level IV procedure in the Royal College of Obstetricians and Gynaecologists classification (the most advanced level of laparoscopic surgery), and can only be performed in highly specialized centers practicing advanced laparoscopic surgery. Laparoscopic uterine nerve ablation, however, should be within the skill of any reasonably competent laparoscopic surgeon practicing in most district general hospitals.

B. Laparoscopic Uterine Nerve Ablation

In 1954, Joseph Doyle from Massachusetts described the procedure of paracervical uterine denervation which bears his name [35]. Doyle's procedure involved the excision of the uterosacral ligaments which carry most of the sensory pain fibers to the lower part of the uterus, at their attachment to the posterior aspect of the cervix. He suggested that the procedure could be performed vaginally by gynecologists, but general surgeons would prefer a large laparotomy incision. His results were extremely impressive, with complete pain relief in 63 out of 73 women (86%), partial relief in 6 cases, and only 4 failures. With such a satisfactory outcome, it is difficult to see why the operation sank into obscurity, but this was possibly due to the advent of the oral contraceptive and prostaglandin synthetase inhibitors (PGSIs), which reduced the demand for such relatively drastic forms of surgical intervention.

In recent years, however, interest in Doyle's procedure has been revived with the advent of minimal access surgery. In addition, the LUNA procedure takes only a few minutes to perform with a surgical laser, electrosurgical needle, or ultrasonic scalpel, and produces the same tissue effect without the need for major surgery. The procedure has an extremely low complication rate.

We have used this procedure as part of our routine treatment for patients with primary dysmenorrhea or secondary dysmenorrhea due to endometriosis for the past 19 years. We have had no serious complications and no increased morbidity over and above diagnostic laparoscopy. Our figures for endometriosis are remarkably similar to those obtained by Joseph Doyle using a laparotomy or vaginal approach to transect the uterosacral ligaments [36] (Table 1).

Laparoscopic uterine nerve ablation can be performed on patients with either primary or secondary dysmenorrhea at the same time as a diagnostic laparoscopy is performed. The pelvis is carefully inspected for associated pathology, particularly endometriosis, and if this is found

Table 1 LUNA Results with CO_2 Laser

	Lost to follow-up	Improved	Same	Worse
Endometriosis, 100 patients	6	81 (86%)	13	—
Primary dysmenorrhea, 26 patients	4	16 (73%)	6	—
Total, 126 patients	10	97 (84%)	19	—

Source: Ref. 36.

the endometriotic implants should be vaporized with the carbon dioxide laser or electrosurgery. The broad ligaments are carefully inspected to try to identify the course of the ureters, which can rarely lie close to the uterosacral ligaments, but are usually 1–2 cm laterally. The characteristic peristaltic movements can usually be recognised beneath the peritoneal surface, but if there is extensive endometriosis with associated fibrosis it is sometimes necessary to dissect out the ureters, which requires considerable laparoscopic surgical expertise.

C. A Critical Appraisal of the Evidence for Laparoscopic Denervation Procedures

A recent Cochrane review [37] suggested that there is insufficient evidence to recommend the use of pelvic neuroablation in the management of dysmenorrhea, regardless of cause. Considering how often the laparoscopic uterine nerve ablation has been performed in recent years, it is surprising that there has been so little in the way of well-designed randomized controlled trials. A small, randomized, double-blind, prospective study was published in 1987 by a team from Detroit [38]. Although there were only 21 patients in this study, it compared LUNA with diagnostic laparoscopy only in patients with primary dysmenorrhea and appeared to be effective in the short term, but its effectiveness appeared to decline over time. Chen et al. [39] confirmed this suggestion and demonstrated that laparoscopic presacral neurectomy may retain its effectiveness for a longer period of time but, as mentioned above, there was a considerable number of unpleasant side effects.

The Guildford Birthright Trial described above had a major flaw in that all patients in the treatment arm had a laparoscopic uterine nerve ablation as well as laser vaporization of all visible endometriotic implants. This inevitably attracted criticism on the basis that there was uncertainty as to which of these procedures contributed to the overall good results. We have recently completed a further randomized, double-blind, prospective trial of 51 patients, in which one group had LUNA plus laser vaporization of endometriosis, while the control arm merely had laparoscopic laser vaporization of endometriosis without any denervation procedure. At 6 months follow-up it was found that the LUNA procedure did not confer any additional benefit on the overall good result, which was almost the same result as in our original randomized, controlled trial [40]. A further study by Vercellini and colleagues came to the same conclusion in a randomized, prospective study with 81 patients [41]. It is interesting to speculate on the overall good results obtained with LUNA in our original retrospective study [42]. A possible explanation is that many patients with severe dysmenorrhea do have deep infiltration of the uterosacral ligaments and the large laser crater (measuring about 2 cm in diameter and 5–10 mm deep) must have clearly removed a lot of this abnormal tissue which is known to give rise to severe pain. We are increasingly seeing young women with deep infiltrating endometriosis running laterally from the rectovaginal septum or a nodule posterior to the cervix, which then infiltrates laterally into the uterosacral ligaments and sometimes even into the pelvic sidewall.

Radical excision of the uterosacral ligaments either with a CO_2 laser or with electrosurgery is increasingly performed, and because the

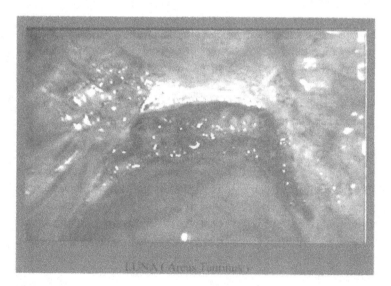

Figure 6   The arcus taurinus procedure. The CO_2 laser vaporization continues laterally to remove all fibromuscular hyperplasia and adenomyosis in the uterosacral ligaments and occasionally has to be extended up the pelvic sidewall if this scar tissue extends to the ureter.

tissue removed is similar to a bull's horn, is called the arcus taurinus (Fig. 6) procedure [43]. Using this technique Jean Bernard Dubuisson and his team in Paris have produced dysmenorrhea relief in 46 out of 50 (92%) women, with dyspareunia relief in 47 out of 51 (92%). They noted that the revised AFS score [15] bore no correlation with symptoms and the scale of disease severity is only really of any value in patients with infertility. They also noticed that the treatment was equally efficacious whether or not the histology showed endometrial glands and stroma. In almost 50% of cases this was not present and the pathological finding was fibromuscular hyperplasia. This observation makes nonsense of the criticism of laser vaporization of the uterosacral ligament disease as being inferior to en bloc dissection because it does not provide a histological specimen. We disagree with this because it the white fibromuscular hyperplasia is clearly visible as one continues vaporizing until one is down to normal tissue. Using this technique, we get similar results to those of other teams using electrosurgery, but our technique takes between 40 min and 1 hr, whereas radical excision can take two or three times this amount of operating time.

D. Ovarian Endometriomas

Ovarian endometriomas, especially those larger than 4 cm in diameter, represent a considerable challenge to laparoscopic surgeons. They are invariably unresponsive to drug treatment, although some shrinkage will occur after aspiration and exposure to GnRH analogues, but unfortunately, once the analogues are discontinued, the endometrioma will reform and continue to increase in size.

They are often associated with deep infiltrating disease of the rectovaginal septum and lateral pelvic sidewall, and are responsible for a considerable amount of pain which classically presents in one or other iliac fossa and radiates through to the lower back and upper buttock. If the endometrioma is stuck to the pelvic sidewall, as is frequently the case, there is often referred pain down the inner or anterior aspect of the thigh, although the pain rarely goes beneath the knee. In some patients, however, the ovarian mass is discovered incidentally and the patient has been completely symptom free, possibly presenting with infertility.

Infertility is usually absolute because of the gross distortion of the tubo-ovarian anatomy, making it impossible for ovum pickup or zygote transport to occur. Nevertheless, although the tubes are grossly hyperemic and swollen, the internal anatomy is usually healthy and the tubes are invariably patent. If the anatomy can be restored to normal, a very gratifying pregnancy rate can be obtained, as well as almost instantaneous pain relief. In our first series of 102 patients with endometriomas from 3 to 20 cm in diameter, 78% of the patients had dramatic pain relief and 57% of those trying to conceive became pregnant, the majority within the first 6 months following the surgery [44]. More recently we reported a further study of 165 women who were randomized to the CO_2 or KTP laser for vaporization of the internal capsule, and noted a slightly lower pregnancy rate of 45% and pain resolution of 74%. There was a much higher recurrence rate of 30% in those patients treated with the CO_2 laser compared with only 12.5% at 1-year follow-up in those treated with the KTP laser [45]. The slightly lower pregnancy rate in this series probably reflects the fact that the CO_2 laser is not the laser of choice in this condition. Endometriomas tend to be very hemorrhagic, and because the CO_2 laser is almost totally absorbed by the water molecule, it does not function as well in these wet conditions as when it is used for vaporization or excision of peritoneal deposits or deep infiltrating disease [46].

If the CO_2 laser is to be used it is better to employ the technique of Donnez [47], in which the endometrioma is aspirated at the first diagnostic laparoscopy or under ultrasound control and then the patients are given a 3-month course of gonadatropin releasing hormone analogues (GnRHa). This not only shrinks the endometrioma, but causes the capsule to be relatively avascular so that the laser can then vaporize the tissue effectively with little damage to the developing follicles underneath.

There is considerable controversy over the pathogenesis of ovarian endometriomas and some authorities consider that they are a completely different disease than peritoneal endometriosis [48]. As long ago as 1957, Hughesden, a gynecological pathologist at University College Hospital in London, suggested that bleeding from endometriotic implants on the posterior surface of the ovary caused the ovary to adhere to the peritoneum of the ovarian fossa, and subsequent bleeding into the space enclosed by the adhesions prevents the escape of the blood and results in invagination of the ovarian cortex as the endometrioma enlarges [49] (Fig. 7). The majority of ovarian endometriomas would appear to fit into this category, because they are densely stuck to the peritoneum of the broad ligament close to the ureter and have to be freed by laparoscopic blunt dissection with a strong stainless steel probe and aqua-dissection, and sometimes need to be divided by laparoscopic scissors. The ovary is gradually levered upward away from the ovarian fossa and during this process it invariably ruptures. The hemosiderin-laden fluid is then aspirated and irrigated until the effluent

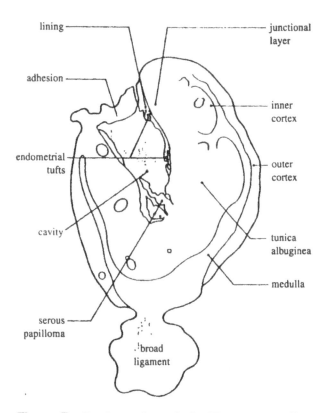

Figure 7 Ovarian endometriosis. The structure of an ovarian endometrioma—a diagrammatic representation. The inside of the chocolate cyst is the outside of the ovarian cortex. (From Ref. 49.)

runs clear, and in our department, the whole of the inside of the endometrioma is photocoagulated with the emerald green KTP/532 laser, which penetrates only a few millimeters and thus causes minimal damage to developing follicles under the surface (Fig. 8). If a KTP/532 laser (Laserscope™ Cwmbran, U.K. and San Jose, CA) is not available, then superficial coagulation can be achieved by using a Bicap™ endocoagulator (Cory Brothers, London, U.K.), which attaches to the suction and irrigation equipment and is relatively simple and safe to use [44,50].

Some laparoscopic surgeons advocate stripping out the ovarian cyst capsule by traction and countertraction. In the case of a true endometrioma, this merely results in stripping out the ovarian cortex and results in profuse bleeding, which requires bipolar coagulation to control, and the inevitable buildup of heat can theoretically result in damage to the developing oocytes beneath the surface. It is important to realize that not all "chocolate cysts" are endometriomas; the chocolate material merely represents hemosiderin and is a reflection of internal

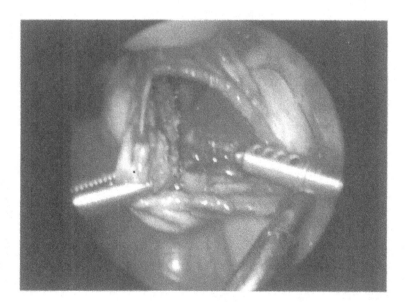

Figure 8 The KTP/532 laser being used to photocoagulate the inside of an endometrioma.

bleeding into the cyst. In most of these situations the ovary is not adherent to the posterior leaf of the broad ligament, but is suspended free from the mesovarium and often represents a benign cystadenoma with internal hemorrhage or a hemorrhagic corpus luteal cyst, or occasionally an endometrioma that has arisen from celomic metaplasia of invaginated epithelial inclusions [51].

However the endometrioma is dealt with by laparoscopic surgery, it is important to be certain at the end of the procedure that there is reasonable hemostasis, and if this is not possible, the ovary can be packed with surgical gauze (Ethicon Endosurgery, Edinburgh, U.K.). On no account should any arterial bleeding be present at the end of the procedure. Sometimes it is tempting to try and restore ovarian anatomy with laparoscopic sutures, but this should be resisted because sutures are a potent cause of tissue ischemia, which is the main initiating factor in adhesion formation [52].

Photocoagulation of the endometrioma capsule with the KTP/532 laser is associated with a low recurrence rate [9]. Daniell from Nashville has reported significant relief of pain and a pregnancy rate of 37.5% in 32 patients trying for conception [50].

Luciano [53] showed that adhesions are more likely to form following laparotomy than laparoscopic surgery. This experimental animal study has been supported in a clinical setting using a randomized trial in which adhesions were assessed at second-look laparoscopy following either laparotomy or laparoscopic surgery in the treatment of tubal pregnancy, and there was much less adhesion formation in the laparoscopy group [54]. Treatment by laparotomy should therefore be resisted, and if facilities, equipment, and technical expertise for laparoscopic surgery are not available, the patient should be referred to centers where these facilities are available.

E. Excision of Capsule or Fenestration and Coagulation

Because there is considerable controversy over the pathogenesis of ovarian endometriomas, it is not surprising that there is equal controversy over the best method of treatment. Those that believe that the Hughesdon hypothesis is the basis for the development of about 90%

of ovarian endometriomas argue that there is no true capsule and one is merely stripping the invaginated ovarian cortex, which is not only difficult, but hemorrhagic, and is more simply treated by coagulation to remove the reddened endometriotic areas to try to prevent recurrence. They further argue that in cases where stripping is easy, the diagnosis is probably wrong and it is more likely to be a follicular hematoma, a hemorrhagic cystadenoma, a hemorrhagic corpus luteum cyst, or even a corpus albicans with hemosiderin deposition [55]. The problem is not just one of comparing like with like, but there are clearly different methods of coagulation available to the laparoscopic surgeon. As mentioned above, we found a considerable difference in the recurrence rate when comparing the KTP laser (12.5%) with the CO_2 laser (30%) when treatment was performed at the same time as the diagnosis was made. Clearly, if the CO_2 laser is the only equipment available for vaporization of the capsule, then in order to obtain good results it is necessary to first aspirate the cyst and then give GnRH analogue therapy for 3 months before the definitive treatment at a second procedure [48].

We have recently performed a prospective, randomized study comparing coagulation of the capsule with the KTP laser at a power setting of 18 W and bipolar coagulation used at a power setting of 70 W. Although the Bicap™ bipolar diathermy equipment is very much less expensive and widely available, we nevertheless found that it was less effective than the KTP laser, and we found that the cyst recurrence rate per patient at 12 months was 21.7% with the Bicap bipolar diathermy compared with only 14.3% with the KTP laser [56].

There is only one prospective, multicenter study comparing laparoscopic cystectomy with drainage and coagulation [57]. This was a cohort study of 366 patients who had a minimum of 6 months follow-up. Six risk factors were evaluated to assess their effect on two separate outcomes. The cumulative rate of cyst recurrence over 48 months was 11.7% and of second surgery was 8.2%. In this study, ultrasonographic cyst recurrence was not associated with pain recurrence in 27.5% of cases. This suggests that if patients are not followed up with serial trans vaginal sonography (TVS) or a second-look laparoscopy, the recurrence rates will be under-reported. In our study, we performed serial postoperative TVS on all our patients and this might explain why our reported recurrence rates appear slightly higher. The stage of the disease in previous surgery for endometriosis was also shown to be an unfavorable prognostic factor.

Patients are increasingly being referred to our unit from other centers with the most severe stages of the disease. In our study, the mean reviewed AFS score was 65.5 (range 22–128) and 75.3% of the patients had stage IV disease. We also found that patients who had recurrent cysts were significantly more likely to have had bilateral cysts compared to single cysts. They were also significantly more likely to have had a previous laparotomy, which required an extensive adhesiolysis and enterolysis before it was possible to treat the endometriomas. When cysts did occur, it was usually in the first 3 months following treatment and this early recurrence is most likely to be the result of incomplete ablation, which in turn may reflect difficulties with access to the cyst.

Tulandi and his team from McGill University in Montreal have presented a retrospective life table analysis, comparing reoperation rates for endometriomas in patients who had undergone laparoscopic treatment by excision and by fenestration [58]. At 12 months the reoperation rates in the two groups were comparable. However, the reoperation rates at 18 months of follow-up were 6.1% after excision and 21.9% after fenestration. This clearly shows that the length of follow-up period is important.

We believe that the KTP laser used at a wavelength of 532 nanometers (which is the same absorption peak as hemosiderin and hemoglobin) is an extremely efficient instrument for photocoagulating the inside of ovarian endometriomas. Our average operating time is of the order of 45 min, in the absence of previous laparotomies, and enables us to do three or four of these cases in a morning operating list. However, the comparison of this technique with excisional stripping of the cyst wall has yet to be examined, and we are in the process of conducting a prospective, randomized multicenter study to try and resolve this issue.

F. Deeply Infiltrating Endometriosis

Deep endometriosis, or adenomyosis [48], is almost invariably located in the rectovaginal septum, the uterosacral ligaments, or sometimes in the uterovesical fold. It can spread laterally up the pelvic side wall causing sclerosis around the ureter, but virtually never infiltrating into the ureter, although it can penetrate into the bladder and large bowel. Deeply infiltrating endometriosis can be associated with the classical or subtle lesions and is often associated with endometriomas of the ovary, but in some women, no endometriosis can be seen laparoscopically, even though the induration can be clearly felt by a combination of rectal and vaginal examination. Colposcopic examination of the vagina often reveals dark blue domed cysts, about 3–4 mm in diameter in the posterior or lateral vaginal fornix. This type of deep infiltrating disease which is virtually unresponsive to drug therapy has to be excised using electrosurgical scissors, needles or ultrasonic scalpels, or vaporized completely with the CO_2 laser until one is down to normal tissue and all the palpable nodules have disappeared. The depth of the lesion has a positive correlation with the amount of pelvic pain [11].

Koninckx [59] has suggested that dioxin and polychlorinated biphenyl pollution is a possible cofactor in the cause and development of deep infiltrating endometriosis, which, in Belgium, is resulting in a steadily increasing proportion of hysterectomies performed for this disease from 10% in 1965 to more than 18% in 1984 [60]. Using epidemiological data reported by the World Health Organisation, they link the highest concentrations of dioxin in breast milk in Belgium [61], which also appears to have the highest incidence of endometriosis in the world, and much of this is of the deeply infiltrating type [62]. The highest concentration of cases is in the industrial corridor running along the south of the country (Donnez J, personal communication, 1998). We should possibly reflect as to whether the obsessive promotion of breastfeeding by our midwives may lead to an epidemic of deep infiltrating endometriosis in industrialized societies.

Dioxin has immunosuppressive activities and is a potent inhibitor of T lymphocyte function [63,64]. A group of rhesus monkeys [65] that were chronically exposed to dioxin for a period of 4 years and followed by serial laparoscopies were found to develop endometriosis 7 years after the termination of dioxin exposure, and in the majority of these cases it was of the deeply infiltrating variety. Dioxin is a potentially harmful by-product of the chlorine-bleaching process used in the wood pulp industry, which includes the manufacture of feminine hygiene products such as tampons. It is worrying that young girls are increasingly being encouraged to use tampons and therefore may be exposing the tissues of the rectovaginal septum and posterior fornix to chronic exposure with a known immunosuppressant. It has been suggested that a woman may use as many as 11,000 tampons in her lifetime and this represents a worrying level of dioxin exposure that could result in deeply infiltrating endometriosis and could explain the increasing incidence of this condition in young women.

G. Surgical Treatment

Before any operative laparoscopy is performed, the patient should have a proctoscopy and sigmoidoscopy or colonoscopy, preferably during menstruation, and appropriate radiological investigations. If the lesion extends laterally, an intravenous urogram is required, but if it is confined to the rectovaginal septum, it is necessary to perform an air-contrast barium enema, sometimes combined with a vaginogram which should be carefully examined in the lateral views by a radiologist experienced in endometriosis management. A thorough bowel preparation is mandatory in all women suspected of having deep endometriosis, and patients should be warned that there is a real risk of perforating the bowel. If perforation occurs, a colorectal surgeon should be available to repair such a defect, although if the bowel preparation has been satisfactory, it should not be necessary to perform a colostomy, and indeed some of the perforations can be adequately repaired transanally or even laparoscopically [66].

In the past it has been necessary to resort to laparotomy for these patients but with increased experience in laparoscopic surgery, many of them can be treated by laparoscopy using CO_2 laser or electrosurgical excision or sharp dissection with scissors. In addition, it is sometimes necessary to perform vaginal excision either from below or by laparoscopy once the plane of cleavage has been developed between the rectum and the vagina [66–69]. Inevitably with this kind of surgery, which is probably the most difficult type of laparoscopic surgery and requires considerable skill and experience, each surgeon will use the method that is best in his or her hands. In our department, we use a high-power ultrapulse CO_2 laser to develop the plane of cleavage between the rectum and the vagina, with special instrumentation to separate these two structures from below and careful palpation in order to avoid damaging the rectum. Even in highly skilled hands such damage is inevitable from time to time. Nezhat [69] reported a series of 174 women in which there were nine bowel perforations and an additional two patients required ureteric stents. Nevertheless, moderate to complete pain relief was achieved in 162 of the women. If dissection has to be very close to the rectum, it is a wise precaution to fill the pelvis with warm Ringer's lactate solution and insufflate the rectum with air or methylene blue to look for any unrecognized rectal lacerations or perforations [66]. A vaginal incision is often (but not routinely) required, and when the vagina is opened, the procedure may be completed vaginally or laparoscopically. In addition, it is sometimes possible to vaporize the vaginal blue-domed cysts via a colposcope with a finger inserted in the rectum to make sure that the vaporization does not damage the rectum.

To excise uterosacral nodules, the peritoneum is incised lateral to the uterosacral ligament. It is necessary to first identify the ureter and occasionally to dissect it out along its course. Once it is displaced laterally, the uterosacral ligament is resected beginning posteriorly and working toward the uterus. Once the nodule has been freed from the underlying tissue the anterior part of the ligament is cut and most of these deep uterosacral implants can be treated without any need for a vaginal incision.

Patients with full-thickness bowel or bladder lesions require more extensive surgery, which is probably better dealt with by laparotomy, although some very advanced laparoscopic surgeons have reported successful results employing transanal circular stapling devices [66] and laparoscopic and transanal or transvaginal repair with or without the help of colorectal surgeons [70,71].

Although this type of surgery is very difficult and time consuming, the results justify the effort, particularly because many of these patients are unresponsive to medical therapy. Koninckx and Martin analyzed their results in 250 women in whom deep endometriosis, had been excised with the CO_2 laser and showed a cure rate of pelvic pain of 70%, with the recurrence rate of less than 5% with a follow-up period up to 5 years [72]. These results should be interpreted with some caution because inevitably there is a learning curve in this kind of surgery. Inspection of the data revealed that the completeness of excision has steadily increased with experience and the results of the recent years strongly suggested an almost complete cure rate with a very low recurrence rate.

H. Pelvic Inflammatory Disease

Pelvic inflammatory disease (PID) is a major public health problem that affects sexually active women worldwide. In spite of the widespread use of antibiotics, it continues to be a major cause of morbidity in women, and some 18–27% of patients presenting with acute pelvic inflammatory disease will develop chronic pelvic pain related to adhesions, hydro/pyosalpinges, and a chronic inflammatory process [73]. A laparoscopy remains the best way of assessing disease severity and of making the diagnosis, and laparoscopic surgery can be used to divide any adhesions and to drain a pyosalpinx by a linear salpingostomy.

The most serious sequelae of pelvic infection is a tubo-ovarian abscess, and despite aggressive treatment with broad spectrum antibiotics, even when accompanied by drainage of pus and excision of the affected organs, it usually results in dense adhesive disease involving the bowel and omentum, causing a syndrome of chronic pelvic pain and infertility. Laparoscopic surgery is best used in the acute phase and uses irrigating fluid under pressure to dissect tissue planes and to gently break down adhesions with blunt dissection. The pus is evacuated, and using toothed ovarian forceps and employing traction and countertraction, the lining exudate of the abscess cavity and all necrotic tissue covering the pelvic organs are gently removed [74]. The procedure requires minimal equipment, but a considerable amount of patience and copious irrigation and suction to remove as much of the infective process as possible. At the end of the procedure, 1 l of warm heparinized Ringer's lactate solution is left in the abdominal cavity to dilute any remaining bacteria and to "aquafloat" the abdominal contents to reduce the chance of subsequent adhesion formation.

The operation is performed under intravenous antibiotic cover and compared to laparotomy, patients recover much more rapidly with less chance of wound infection, decreased risk of bowel perforation, and a more thorough removal of pus and nectrotic material from the pelvic cavity.

In our experience, second-look laparoscopy 6 weeks to 3 months later reveals a remarkably normal looking pelvis, and any de novo adhesions can easily be dissected from their origin and attachment by laparoscopic scissor dissection, but in practice this is rarely necessary.

Up to 15% of women with laparoscopically proven pelvic inflammatory disease have evidence of perihepatitis and develop fibrinous adhesions rather like violin strings between the liver surface and the diaphragm and anterolateral abdominal wall. This condition, the Fitz-Hugh-Curtis syndrome, was first described following gonococcal infection, but is most frequently seen in women with chlamydial trachomatis PID [75]. Patients complain of pain in the right upper quadrant of the abdomen which can mimic cholecystitis, and in 50% of patients bilirubin and serum enzymes are mildly elevated [76]. These adhesions can easily be divided through appropriately placed ports using laparoscopic scissors, a carbon dioxide laser with a backstop probe, or a KTP laser fiber with very satisfactory symptom relief.

I. Adhesions

Adhesion formation has always been one of the most regrettable aftermaths of surgery, particularly fertility surgery, where adhesion formation can interfere with ovum pickup and transport of the fertilized oocyte. There is, however, considerable controversy as to whether intra-abdominal adhesions are causally related to pelvic pain. Several workers have drawn attention to the type of adhesion that restricts the mobility or distensibility of the pelvic and abdominal wall organs, particularly the bowel [77,78]. It has also been shown that the location of the pain is in the area of the adhesions in 90% of women, although there is no correlation between the severity of the pain and the extent of the adhesions [79]. Conscious pain mapping in one study showed that 25 of 31 (80.6%) women with adhesions reported tenderness on manipulation of these adhesions under conscious sedation (fentanyl) [80]. Another possible mechanism of pain, which possibly explains this, is the fact that some adhesions are not only vascularized but also develop a nerve supply. Kligman et al. took adhesions from 17 patients, 10 of whom had chronic pelvic pain and 7 who were pain free. There was evidence of nerve fibers in 10 of these adhesions, but they were evenly distributed between the two groups [81]. In 1990, we reported a study in our department [82] of a group of 118 women who were followed between 1 and 5 years, in whom the site of adhesion appeared to correlate with the location of the pain. Most of the adhesions were due to previous surgery and in offending order were the operations of appendectomy, reconstructive surgery on the ovaries at laparotomy (including patients who had microsurgery), operations for ectopic pregnancy, and caesarean section. In this group of patients, 84 (76%) were completely better with no further pain. In 7 patients their symptoms had improved but were still present, and a further 19 patients showed no improvement at all. Eight of these patients were lost to follow-up, but in all cases the laparoscopic surgery had been uneventful without complications and all had returned to work or full domestic activity within 48 hrs of the laparoscopic laser adhesiolysis. The type of adhesions that we were dealing with were not the loose floppy omental adhesions, which one often sees during a laparoscopy in patients who have had previous surgery, but were a tight band of adhesions that were impairing the motility of a loop of bowel (Fig. 9).

When we had completed the study we were interested to see a leading article in the *British Medical Journal* by a distinguished general surgeon from Birmingham, U.K., John Alexander Williams, entitled "Do Adhesions Cause Pain?" His conclusion was "I believe it to be a poorly substantiated myth that adhesions can cause abdominal or pelvic pain." It must be remembered that this was before surgeons were doing laparoscopic surgery for cholecystectomy and before they were involved in enterolysis procedures. This was, therefore, not an entirely unreasonable statement because at that time surgeons undertaking adhesiolysis procedures were always doing it by laparotomy, which has a high incidence of adhesion reformation, as has been shown in many studies [83]. Clearly Williams realized that any operation to remove the adhesions would be more likely to result in further adhesion formation. Since laparoscopic surgery has been widely accepted by our surgical colleagues, they are much more likely to attempt quite difficult enterolysis procedures, and because they are more adequately qualified to deal with any problems encountered with bowel adhesions, I now

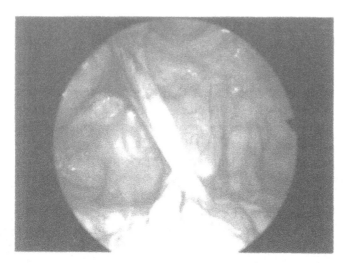

Figure 9   Tight adhesive band impairing the motility of the small bowel at
the site of maximum pain.

tend to allow them to do this kind of surgery in severe cases. Although
we perform a great deal of enterolysis procedures, we nowadays would
tend to use scissors rather than the CO_2 laser. However, in 1990 the
scissors that were available were of a very poor quality, reusable, and
were not self sharpening; this was the reason that we preferred the
cutting ability of the CO_2 laser. With the introduction of sharp, dispos-
able scissors, the laser would now be a much more complicated way
of dealing with this problem.

The relationship of adhesions to pelvic pain is by no means clear-
cut. The study of Kresch [77], which compared 100 women with
chronic pelvic pain to another group of asymptomatic patients having
laparoscopic sterilization, showed that in the pain group 38% had adhesions and 32% had endometriosis, compared with 12% having adhesions and 15% having endometriosis in the study group. Their conclusion, like ours, was that the adhesions in the patients with chronic
pelvic pain were more likely to be due to restriction of bowel, particularly loops of small bowel. They had to admit, however, that adhesions
in women with chronic pelvic pain with no associated pelvic pathology
were not consistently associated with pain, and a further study by How-

ard [84] concluded that women with adhesions complained of chronic pelvic pain in 25% of cases, but 17% of those with no pain also had adhesions. Another study by Peters [78] concluded that patients with severe adhesions have better long-term pain relief than those with lesser degrees of adhesion formation, and that severe adhesions were more likely to be associated with chronic pelvic pain. Our own study [82] agreed with the findings of Kresch et al. [77] that adhesions restricting distension and movement of the pelvic organs, particularly the bowel, are more likely to be associated with chronic pelvic pain.

Research has suggested that a reduction in mesothelial plasminogen activator activity in the presence of trauma, infection or tissue ischemia is the likely pathway in post-surgical adhesion formation [85–87]. Unfortunately, application of plasminogen activator is not particularly effective, so we irrigate with 4% icodextrin and try to leave a liter in the pelvis. This remains for about 7 days, separating the traumatized surfaces and allowing them to heal without adhering to each other. Icodextrin (Adept™ ML Laboratories, Liverpool, U.K.) is a large molecule which has been used for many years in peritoneal dialysis. It is broken down by amylase and because there is normally no amylase in the peritoneal cavity, it remains for about 1 week. At present, there are no controlled trials on the efficacy of this adhesion barrier, but initial experience in our department shows that it is easy to use. It is hoped that some second-look data will be available soon.

VI. OTHER LESS COMMON CAUSES OF PELVIC PAIN

A. Ovarian Tumors

Ovarian tumors can present with pelvic pain as a result of intracystic hemorrhage, cyst rupture or, rarely, ovarian torsion. In a study of laparoscopic findings in women with chronic pelvic pain by Porpora and Gomel from Rome and Vancouver, they accounted for 16% of the cases if endometriomas were excluded [88]. As long as the ovarian lesions are not too large, they can nearly always be treated by laparoscopic surgery, either by fenestration, aspiration, and coagulation of the cyst lining after suitable biopsies have been taken, or by excision of the cyst capsule with an attempt to preserve as much normal ovary as possible. Great care should be taken in the preoperative assessment by color Doppler ultrasound performed by an ultrasonologist experienced in ovarian scanning, and even if this is reassuring, the intra-operative inspection of the entire abdominal and pelvic cavity, with the appropriate washings and biopsies, should always be undertaken to exclude malignancy.

B. Uterine Retroversion

Uterine retroversion can be associated with deep dyspareunia owing to the proximity of the ovaries to the top of the vagina when the uterus is in this position. It can also be associated with chronic pelvic pain, congestive dysmenorrhea, and may give rise to backache.

Laparoscopic ventrosuspension was one of the earlier laparoscopic operations and was first reported in the English-language literature by Patrick Steptoe in his monologue on laparoscopy, which he wrote after visiting Raoul Palmer in Paris. The procedure appears to be performed less often nowadays, and this is possibly due to the fact that shortening of the round ligaments and suturing them into the rectus sheath can be quite painful postoperatively and there is always a risk of distortion of the fallopian tube. In addition, the remaining part of the round ligaments often stretch again during the following year. Yoong [89] reported 72 patients treated by laparoscopic ventrosuspension and only 51.5% had reduction of pain following the procedure, and this decreased to 46.5% at 6 months. Raslan et al., however, reported an 81% reduction of deep dyspareunia and a 76% improvement in pelvic pain 1 year after the operation [90].

C. Pelvic Congestion Syndrome

Not infrequently one finds no obvious cause for pelvic pain, apart from marked varicosities in the parametrium and often in the ovarian venous plexus. These can be made to stand out if the patient is flattened during inspection of the pelvis, although an additional probe will be necessary to keep the bowel from obscuring laparoscopic vision. The diagnosis can be confirmed with pelvic venography or by transvaginal ultrasound using color Doppler to demonstrate distended veins. These patients often have deep dyspareunia, congestive dysmenorrhea and post-coital ache, and various other sexual problems. They constitute a difficult group of women to treat and often have marital and sexual problems, psychological disturbances and, frequently, a history of sexual abuse when they were young [91]. Attempts have been made to ligate the ovarian vein laparoscopically, but there is often a large number of vessels involved and to be effective, it needs to be done high up above the pelvic brim, which should only really be undertaken by surgeons with advanced laparoscopic skills and experience with laparoscopic aortic lymphadenectomy. In a small series of patients embolization has been shown to be effective [92].

Attempts at medical treatment or psychotherapy often yield disappointing results, and many of these women eventually come to hysterectomy with or without bilateral oophorectomy. Stovall et al. [93] studied a group of women who had hysterectomy for chronic pelvic pain without any preoperative evidence of pelvic disease and found that 35% of the 99 women were found to have either adenomyosis or fibroids. Two years after the procedure, 78% of the patients remained well, but 22% had persisting pain.

It seems that, as with endometriosis, laparoscopy offers a great deal of hope for many sufferers of chronic pelvic pain and its various manifestations, but there will always remain a number of women who appear to fail to respond to any conventionally available therapy at present.

REFERENCES

1. Mathias SD, Kupperman M, Liberman RF, et al. Chronic pelvic pain: prevalence, health-related quality of life and economic correlates. Obstet Gynecol 1996; 87:321–327.
2. Porpora MG, Gomel V. The role of laparoscopy in the management of pelvic pain in women of reproductive age. Fertil Steril 1997; 68:765–779.
3. Vercellini P, Fedele L, Molteni P, Arcaini L, Bianci S, Candiani GB. Laparoscopy in the diagnosis of gynaecological chronic pelvic pain. Int J Gynaecol Obstet 1990; 32:261–265.

4. Contoravdis A, Chryssikopoulos A, Hassiakos D, et al. The diagnostic value of laparoscopy in 2365 patients with acute and chronic pelvic pain. Int J Gynaecol Obstet 1996; 52:243–248.

5. Howard FM. Laparoscopic evaluation and treatment of women with chronic pelvic pain. J Am Gynaecol Lapro 1994; 1:325–331.

6. Newham AP, van der Spuy ZM, Nugent F. Laparoscopic findings in women with chronic pelvic pain. S Afr Med J 1996; 86:1200–1203.

7. Wiborny R, Pichler B. Endoscopic dissection of the uterosacral ligaments for treatment of chronic pelvic pain. Gynaecol Endosc 1998; 7: 33–35.

8. O'Connor D. Endometriosis. In: Singer A, Jordan JA, eds. Current Reviews in Obstetrics and Gynaecology. Edinburgh: Churchill Livingstone, 1987.

9. Mahmood TA, Templeton AA, Thompson L, Fraser C. Menstrual symptoms in women with pelvic endometriosis. Br J Obstet Gynaecol 1991; 98:558–563.

10. Vernon MW, Beard JS, Graves K, Wilson EA. Classification of endometriotic implants by morphological appearance and capacity to synthesise prostaglandin F. Fertil Steril 1986; 46:801–806.

11. Cornillie FJ, Oosterlynck D, Sauweryns J, Koninckx PR. Deep infiltrating pelvic endometriosis: histology and clinical significance. Fertil Steril 1993; 53:978–983.

12. Sutton CJG. In: Phipps J, ed. Laparoscopy and the Adnexal Mass. Endometriosis. Infertility and Reproductive Medicine in Clinics of North America 1995; 6:591–613.

13. Nisolle M, Donnez J. Peritoneal endometriosis, ovarian endometriosis and adenomyotic nodules of the recto-vaginal septum are three different entities. Fertil Steril 1997; 68:585–596.

14. Koninckx PS, Martin DC. Deep endometriosis: a consequence of infiltration or retraction or possibly adenomyosis externa? Fertil Steril 1992; 58:924–928.

15. The American Fertility Society. Revised American Fertility Society classification of endometriosis: 1985. Fertil Steril 1985; 43:351–352.

16. Sutton CJG, Nair S, Ewen SP, Haines P. A comparison between the CO_2 and KTP lasers in the treatment of large ovarian endometriomas. Gynaecol Endosc 1993; 2:113.

17. Revill SI, Robinson JO, Rosen M, Hogg MIJ. The reliability of a linear analogue scale for evaluating pain. Anaesthesia 1976; 31:1191–1196.

18. Sutton CJG, Hill D. Laser laparoscopy in the treatment of endometriosis. A 5-year study. Br J Obstet Gynaecol 1990; 97:181–185.

19. Fedele L, Bianchi S, Bocciolone L, Di Nola G, Franchi D. Buserelin acetate in the management of pelvic pain associated with minimal and mild endometriosis: a controlled study. Fertil Steril 1993; 59:516–521.

20. Sutton CJG, Pooley AS, Ewen SP, Haines P. Follow-up report on randomised controlled trial of laser laparoscopy in the treatment of pelvic pain associated with minimal to moderate endometriosis. Fertil Steril 1997; 68:1070–1074.

21. D'Hooghe TM. Natural history of endometriosis in baboons: is endometriosis an intermittent and/or progressive disease? In: Venturini PL, Evers JLH, eds. Endometriosis: Basic Research & Clinical Practice. Carnforth, U.K.: Parthenon Publishing, 1998:51–58.

22. Jones KD, Sutton C, Haines P. A long-term follow-up report on controlled trial of laser laparoscopy for pelvic pain. J Soc Laparoendosc Surg 2001; 10:217–222.

23. Sutton CJG, Dover RW, Pooley A, Jones K, Haines P. Prospective, randomised, double-blind controlled trial of laparoscopic laser uterine nerve ablation in the treatment of pelvic pain associated with endometriosis. Gynaecol Endosc 2001. In press.

24. Johnson N, Wilson M, Farquhar C. Surgical pelvic neuro-ablation for chronic pelvic pain: a systematic review. Gynaecol Endosc 2000; 9:351–361.

25. Owman C, Rosenbren E, Sjoberg NO. Adrenergic innovation of the human female reproductive organs: a histochemical and chemical investigation. Obstet Gynaecol 1967; 30:763–773.

26. Frankenhäuser G. Die Bewegungenerven der Gebarmutter. Z Med Nat Wiss 1864; 1:35–39.

27. Campbell RM. Anatomy & physiology of sacro-uterine ligaments. Am J Obstet Gynecol 1950; 59:1–5.

28. Latarjet A, Roget P. Le plexus hypogastrique chez la femme. Gynaecol Obstet 1922; 6:225–228.

29. Cotte G. Resection of the presacral nerve in the treatment of obstinate dysmenorrhoea. Am J Obstet Gynaecol 1937; 33:1034–1040.

30. Biggerstaff ED. Laparoscopic surgery for pelvic pain. In: Sutton CJG, Diamond M, eds. Endoscopic Surgery for Gynaecologists, 2nd ed. London: W.B. Saunders, 1998:261–271.

31. Daniell JF, Lalonde CJ. Advanced laparoscopic procedures for pelvic pain and dysmenorrhoea. In: Sutton CJG, ed. Clinical Obstetrics and Gynaecology Advanced Laparoscopic Surgery. London: Bailliere Tindall, 1995; 9:795–807.

32. Nezhat C, Nezhat F. A simplified method of laparoscopic pre-sacral neu-

rectomy for the treatment of central pelvic pain due to endometriosis. Br J Obstet Gynaecol 1992; 99:659–663.

33. Chen FP, Chang SD, Chu KK, Soong YK. Comparison of laparoscopic pre-sacral neurectomy and laparoscopic uterine nerve ablation for primary dysmenorrhoea. J Reprod Med 1996; 41:463–466.

34. Candiani GB, Fedele L, Vercellini P, Bianchi S, Di Nola G. Presacral neurectomy for the treatment of pelvic pain associated with endometriosis: a controlled study. Am J Obstet Gynecol 1992; 167:100–103.

35. Doyle JB. Paracervical uterine denervation for dysmenorrhoea. Trans. New Engl Obst Gynec Soc 1954; 8:143–146.

36. Sutton C. Laparoscopic uterine nerve ablation for intractable dysmenorrhoea. In: Sutton C, Diamond M. Endoscopic Surgery for Gynaecologists, 2nd ed. London: W.B. Saunders, 1998:249–260.

37. Johnson N, Wilson M, Farquhar C. Surgical pelvic neuroablation for chronic pelvic pain: a systematic review. Gynaecol Endosc 2000; 9:351–341.

38. Lichten EM, Bombard J. Surgical treatment of primary dysmenorrhoea with laparoscopic uterine nerve ablation. J Reprod Med 1987; 32:37–41.

39. Chen FP, Chang SD, Chu KK, Soong YK. Comparison of laparoscopic Pre-sacral neurectomy and laparoscopic uterine nerve ablation for primary dysmenorrhoea. J Reprod Med 1996; 41:463–466.

40. Sutton CJG, Dover RW, Pooley A, Jones K, Haines P. Prospective, randomised, double-blind controlled trial of laparoscopic laser uterine nerve ablation in the treatment of pelvic pain associated with endometriosis. Gynaecol Endosc 2001; 10:217–222.

41. Vercellini P, Aimi G, Busacca M, Uglietti A, Viganali M, Crossignani PG. Laparoscopic uterosacral ligament resection for dysmenorrhoea associated with endometriosis: Results of a randomised controlled trial (abstr). Fertil Steril 1997; 68(suppl 1):3.

42. Sutton CJG. Laser uterine nerve ablation. In: Donnez J, Nisolle M, eds. An Atlas of Laser Operative Laparoscopy and Hysteroscopy. Louvan, Belgium: Nauerwelaerts Publishing 1994:47–52.

43. Jones KD, Sutton C. Arcus taurinus: 'the mother and father' of all LUNAs. Review article. Gynaecol Endosc 2001; 10:83–89.

44. Sutton CJG. Lasers in infertility. Hum Reprod 1993; 8:133–146.

45. Sutton CJG, Ewen SP, Jacobs SA, Whitelaw N. Laser laparoscopic surgery in the treatment of ovarian endometriomas. J Am Assoc Gynecol Laparosc 1997; 4:319–323.

46. Sutton CJG, Hodgson R. Endoscopic cutting with lasers. Minim Invasive Ther 1992; 1:197–205.

47. Donnez J, Nisolle M, Gillet N, Smets M, Bassil S, Casanas-Roux F. Large ovarian endometriomas. Hum Reprod 1996; 11:641–646.
48. Nisolle M. Peritoneal ovarian and recto-vaginal endometriosis are three distinct entities. These d'Agregation de l'enseignement Superieur, Universite Catholique de Louvain, Louvain, Belgium. 1996.
49. Hughesdon PE. The structure of endometrial cysts of the ovary. J Obstet Gynaecol Br Emp 1957; 44:69–84.
50. Daniell JF, Kurtz BR, Gurley LD. Laser laparoscopic management of large endometriomas. Fertil Steril 1991; 55:692–695.
51. Donnez J, Nisolle M, Casanas-Roux F, Clerks F. Endometriosis: rationale for surgery. In: Brosen I, Donnez J, eds. Current State of Endometriosis. Research and Management. Carnforth: Parthenon Publishing, 1993: 385–395.
52. Rafftery A. The effect of peritoneal trauma on peritoneal fibrinolytic activity and intraperitoneal adhesion formation. Eur Surg Res 1981; 13: 397–401.
53. Luciano AA, Maier D, Coch E, Nillsen J, Whitman F. A comparative study of post-operative adhesions following laser surgery by laparoscopy versus laparotomy in the rabbit model. Obstet Gynecol 1989; 74:220–224.
54. Lundorff P, Hahlin M, Kiallfelt B, Thorburn J, Lindblom B. Adhesion formation after laparoscopic surgery in tubal pregnancy: a randomised trial versus laparotomy. Fertil Steril 1991; 55:911–915.
55. Sutton CJG. Endometriosis. In: Phipps JH, ed. Infertility and Reproductive Medicine. Clinics of North America. Adnexal masses. Philadelphia: W.B. Saunders, 1995; (6)3:591–613.
56. Jones KD, Sutton CJG. Laparoscopic surgery for endometriosis. Abstract presented at The British Congress of Obstetrics and Gynaecology, Birmingham, UK, July 2001. Conference Abstracts, RCOG Publications, Royal College of Obstetricians and Gynaecologist, London, U.K.
57. Beretta P, Franchi M, Ghezzi F, Busacca M, Zupi E, Bolis P. Randomised clinical trial of two laparoscopic treatments of endometriomas: cystectomy versus drainage and coagulation. Fertil Steril 1998; 70:1176–1180.
58. Saleh A, Tulandi T. Re-operation after laparoscopic treatment of endometriomas by excision and fenestration. Fertil Steril 1999; 72:322–324.
59. Koninckx PR, Braet P, Kennedy S, Barlow DH. Dioxin pollution and endometriosis in Belgium. Hum Reprod 1994; 9:1001–1002.
60. National Centre for Health Statistics. Hysterectomies in the United States. 1965–84. Vital and Health statistics. Data from the National

Health Survey; 1987. Hyattsville, MD: National Centre for Health Statistics, Series 13, No. 92, DHSS Publ. (PHS) 88–175.

61. World Health Organisation. Level of PCB's, PCDD's and PCDF's in breast milk: result of WHO co-ordinated interlaboratory quality control studies and analytical field studies. WHO Environmental Health Series, Geneva, 1989.

62. Martin DC, Hubert GD, Van der Zwaag R, El Zeky FA. Laparoscopic appearances of peritoneal endometriosis. Fertil Steril 1989; 51:63–67.

63. Holsapple MP, Snyder NK, Wood SC, Morris DL. A review of 2,3,7,8-tetrachlorodibenzo-p-dioxin-induced changes in immunocompetence. Toxicology 1991; 69:219–255.

64. Neubert R, Jacob-Muller U, Stahlmann R, Helge H, Neubert D. Polyhalogenated dibenzo-p-dioxins and dibenzofurans and the immune system. Arch Toxicol 1992; 65:213–219.

65. Rier SE, Martin DC, Bowman RE, Dmowsky WP, and Becker JL. Endometriosis in rhesus monkeys (Macaca mulatta) following chronic exposure to 2,3,7,8-tetrachlorodibenzo-p-dioxin. Fundam Appl Toxicol 1993; 21:433–441.

66. Reich H, McGlynn F, Salvat J. Laparoscopic treatment of cul-de-sac obliteration secondary to retrocervical deep fibrotic endometriosis. J Reprod Med 1991; 3:516–522.

67. Martin DC. Laparoscopic treatment of advanced endometriosis. In: Sutton CJG, Diamond M, eds. Endoscopic Surgery for Gynaecologists. London: W.B. Saunders, 1993:229–237.

68. Martin DC. Laparoscopic and vaginal colpotomy for the excision of infiltrating cul-de-sac endometriosis. J Reprod Med Obstet Gynaecol 1988; 33:806–808.

69. Nezhat C, Nezhat F, Pennington E. Laparoscopic treatment of infiltrative rectosigmoid colon and rectovaginal septum endometriosis by the technique of video laparoscopy and the CO_2 laser. Br J Obstet Gynaecol 1992; 99:664–667.

70. Redwine DB. Non-laser resection of endometriosis. In: Sutton CJG, Diamond M, eds. Endoscopic Surgery for Gynaecologists. London: W.B. Saunders, 1993:220–228.

71. Redwine DB, Sharpe DR. Laparoscopic segmental resection of the sigmoid colon for endometriosis. J Laparoendoscop Surg 1991; 1:217–220.

72. Koninckx PR, Martin DC. Treatment of deeply infiltrating endometriosis. In: Sutton CJG, ed. Gynaecologic Surgery and Endoscopy. Current Opinion in Obstetrics and Gynaecology. Hagerstown: Lippincott, Williams & Wilkins, 1994:231–241.

73. Goldstein DP, De Choinoky C, Emans SJ, Leventhal JM. Laparoscopy in the diagnosis and management of pelvic pain in adolescence. J Reprod Med 1980; 24:251–256.

74. Reich H, McGlynn F. Laparoscopic treatment of tubo-ovarian and pelvic abscess. J Reprod Med 1989; 32:747–749.

75. Eschenbach DA, Wolner-Hansson P. Fitz-Hugh Curtis syndrome. In: Holmes KK, Mardh PA, Sparling PF, Wiesner PJ, eds. Sexually Transmitted Diseases. New York: McGraw-Hill, Inc., 1990:621–626.

76. Bevan C. Pelvic inflammatory disease. Clinical Guidelines 126, 1998. Royal College of Obstetricians and Gynaecologists, London.

77. Kresch AJ, Seifer DB, Sachs LB, Barrese I. Laparoscopy in 100 women with chronic pelvic pain. Obstet Gynecol 1984; 64:672–674.

78. Peters AAW, Trimbos-Kemper GCM, Admiral C, Trimbos JB. A randomised clinical trial on the benefit of adhesiolysis in patients with intraperitoneal adhesions and chronic pelvic pain. Br J Obstet Gynaecol 1992; 99:59–62.

79. Stout AL, Steege JF, Dodson WC, Hughes CL Relationship of laparoscopic findings to self report of pelvic pain. Am J Obstet Gynecol 1991; 164:73–79.

80. Almeida OD, Val-Gallas JM. Conscious pain mapping. J Am Assoc Gynecol Laparosc 1997; 4:587–590.

81. Kligman I, Drachenberg C, Papadimitriou J, Katz E. Immuno-histochemical demonstration of nerve fibres in pelvic adhesions. Obstet Gynaecol 1993; 82:566–568.

82. Sutton C, MacDonald R. Laser laparoscopic adhesiolysis. J Gynaecol Surg 1990; 6:155–159.

83. Luciano AA, Maier D, Coch E, Nillsen J, Whitman F. A comparative study of post-operative adhesions following laser surgery by laparoscopy versus laparotomy in the rabbit model. Obstet Gynecol 1989; 74:220–224.

84. Howard FM The role of laparoscopy in chronic pelvic pain—promise and pitfalls. Obstet Gynaecol Surg 1993; 48:357–387.

85. Buckman RF, Woods M, Sargent L, Gervin AS. A unifying pathogenic mechanism in the aetiology of intra-peritoneal adhesions. J Surg Res 1976; 20:1–5.

86. Raftery AT. Effect of peritoneal trauma on peritoneal fibrinolytic activity and intraperitoneal adhesion formation. An experimental study in the rat. Eur Surg Res 1981; 13:397–401.

87. Menzies D, Ellis H. Intra-abdominal adhesions and their prevention by topical tissue plasminogen activator. J R Soc Med 1989; 82:534–535.

88. Porpora MG, Gomel V. The role of laparoscopy in the management of pelvic pain in women of reproductive age. Fertil Steril 1997; 68:765–779.

89. Yoong AF. Laparoscopic ventrosuspension. A review of 72 cases. Am J Obstet Gynecol 1990; 163:1151–1153.

90. Raslan F, Lynch CB, Rix J. Symptoms relieved by endoscopic ventrosuspension. Gynaecol Endosc 1995; 4:101–104.

91. Reiter RC, Shakerin LR, Gambone JC, Milburn AK. Correlation between sexual abuse and somatisation in women with somatic and nonsomatic chronic pelvic pain. Am J Obstet Gynecol 1991; 165:104–109.

92. Sichlau MJ, Yao JS, Bogelzac RL. Transcatheter embolotherapy for the treatment of pelvic congestion syndrome. Obstet Gynecol 1994; 82:892–896.

93. Stovall TG, Ling FW, Crawford DA. Hysterectomy for chronic pelvic pain of presumed uterine aetiology. Obstet Gynecol 1990; 95:676–679.

Index

Adhesions, 272
Anabolic therapy, 84
Androgen, 39 androgen and bone, 45, 46
Antibiotics and oral contraceptive pills, 16
Antiresorptive therapy, 84

Biphosphonates, 85, 92
Bone mineral density, 82
Brain, 51
Breast cancer, 13, 50, 62, 65

Calcitonin, 94
Calcium, 89
Cancer, 57
Cardiovascular effects, 11
Cervical cancer, 67, 68
Chromosome:
  abnormality, 137
  aneuploidy, 139
  autosomal dominant, 146

[Chromosome]
  autosomal recessive, 141
  translocations, 139
  X-linked, 149
Colorectal cancer, 70
Condom, 9
Contraception:
  adverse effects, 28
  barrier, 9
  benefits, 25, 26
  contraceptive patch, 8
  failure rates, 5, 25
  implants, 7
  injectable, 8
  mechanism, 23
  oral contraception 6
  progestin-only, 10
  ultralow-dose, 23
Cryobiology, 167
Cryopreservation:
  cryoprotectant, 173
  fertilization, 181

[Cryopreservation]
 oocyte, 167
 ovarian tissue, 183
 pregnancy, 181
 program, 175
 safety, 184
 slow freezing, 175
 survival rate, 180
 timing, 179
 vitrification,176

Diabetes, 10, 32
Diaphragm, 9

Ectopic pregnancy:
 diagnosis, 225, 228
 expectant treatment, 238
 hCG, 227, 229
 laparoscopy, 228, 235
 methotrexate, 230, 231
 persistent, 239
 reproductive performance,
  240
 salpingectomy, 236
 salpingostomy, 236, 237, 238
 surgical treatment, 234
 symptoms, 225
 ultrasound, 226, 229
Embryo:
 development, 120
 transfer, 120
Endometrial cancer, 58, 61
Endometrium, 50, 58
Endometriosis:
 deep, 267
 endometrioma, 261
 laparoscopy, 246, 269
Endometrioma:
 excision, 265

[Endometrioma]
 fenestration, 265
 treatment, 261
Epilepsy and contraception, 14

Fecundity, 2,3
Fertility, 2, 3
FISH, 138
Fluoride, 85, 95
Fracture, 44

Growth factor and bone turnover,
  86
Growth hormone, 98

Hormonal replacement therapy
 (HRT), 39, 57
Hot flushes, 43
Hypertension, 12

Intrauterine device, 8
In vitro fertilization, 111
In vitro maturation, 109

Lactating, 34
Laparoscopy:
 denervation, 256
 ectopic pregnancy, 235
 endometriosis, 246
 laser, 248
 pelvic pain, 245
 presacral neurectomy, 256
 uterine nerve ablation, 257,
  259
Leiomyoma, 34
Lipids, 11, 31, 48

Methotrexate:
 local, 233
 monitoring, 232

[Methotrexate]
multidose, 232
side effects, 231
treatment, 230, 231
Migraine, 13, 32
Mood, 43

Oocytes:
cryopreservation, 165
donation, 124
fertilization, 119
immature, 178, 183
in vitro maturation, 110,
118
maturation, 109
retrieval, 115
selection for cryopreservation,
177
Ovary:
normal, 122
polycystic, 111
Osteopenia, 83
Osteoporosis, 12, 44, 81
diagnosis, 82
pathophysiology, 82
Ovarian cancer, 69, 70

Parathyroid hormone, 96, 98
Pelvic pain:
laparoscopy, 245
ovarian tumors, 275
Pelvic inflammatory disease,
271
Pelvic congestion, 276
Preimplantation genetic diagnosis:
allele drop-out, 151
and FISH, 138
approaches, 135

contamination, 150
techniques, 141
PTH, 96

Seizure disorder and contraception,
14, 33
Selective estrogen receptor modula-
tor, 64, 85, 89
SERMs, 64, 85, 89
Sex selection, 136
Sexuality, 40, 41
Sickle cell, 13, 33
Sterilization, 4

Testosterone, 41
Thyroid, 17
Thyroid cancer, 71

Uterus:
anomaly, 195
normal development, 198
retroverted, 276
Uterine anomaly:
agenesis, 203
arcuate, 216
bicornuate, 212
classification, 195
DES related, 216
diagnosis, 196, 200
didelphys, 211
impact on fertility, 199
impact on obstetric function,
199
incidence, 198
septate, 213
unicornuate, 208

Vasomotor symptoms, 43
Vitamin D, 85, 89